Birth Trap

THE LEGAL LOW-DOWN ON HIGH-TECH OBSTETRICS

Birth Trap

THE LEGAL LOW-DOWN
ON HIGH-TECH OBSTETRICS

YVONNE BRACKBILL, Ph.D.

Graduate Research Professor,
University of Florida, Gainesville, Florida;
Member/Fellow, International Childbirth Education Association;
InterNational Association of Parents and Professionals
for Safe Alternatives in Childbirth

JUNE RICE, B.A., M.P.A., J.D.

Assistant Public Defender,
Key West, Florida

DIONY YOUNG, B.A.

Consultant, International Childbirth Education Association;
New York State Prenatal-Perinatal Advisory Council

Forewords by

Robert S. Mendelsohn, M.D.

Richard E. Hartman, Esquire

The C. V. Mosby Company

ST. LOUIS • NEW YORK • TORONTO   1984

Editor: Nancy L. Mullins
Manuscript editor: Margaret A. Weeter
Design: Diane M. Beasley
Production: Margaret B. Bridenbaugh

Printed in the United States of America

THE MOSBY PRESS
The C.V. Mosby Company
11830 Westline Industrial Drive, St. Louis, Missouri 63146

Library of Congress Cataloging in Publication Data

Brackbill, Yvonne.
  Birth trap.

  Bibliography: p.
  Includes index.
  1. Childbirth. 2. Pregnant women—Legal status, laws, etc.—United States. 3. Obstetricians—Malpractice. 4. Childbirth—Social aspects. I. Rice, June. II. Young, Diony, 1938-   . III. Title.
RG652.B69 1984   346.7303'32   84-3487
ISBN 0-8016-0678-0   347.306332

F/D/D 9 8 7 6 5 4 3 2 1   03/B/335

To the
7,000,000 American men and women who will become parents this year,
and to the
7,000,000 who will become parents next year,
and to the
7,000,000 who will become parents each year after that.

Acknowledgments

The guidance and support of many people—family, friends, colleagues, and clients—are important in the production of any major undertaking. This is true in the writing of this book. We thank all who have helped us crystallize our thinking by sharing their personal experiences and knowledge. We must extend special thanks to Nikki Archer, Beverley Beech, Jamie Bolane, Eunice K. Ernst, Doris Haire, C.C. Hopkins, John Roscow III, David Stewart, and Melva Weber.

Foreword

Of the hundreds of books written in the past decade on childbirth, this one stands out as the most important.

Its title points to the most powerful weapon ever available to women facing the carnage of modern obstetrics. Indeed, Yvonne Brackbill, June Rice, and Diony Young have supplied every American citizen the ammunition necessary to torpedo the juggernaut of hospital deliveries.

No hearts and flowers, sweet, soft music of home births here. No exaggeration, no hyperbole, no hard sell, no hype. Instead, hard data, cold facts, objective presentation, impeccable documentation fill this book by America's most credentialized childbirth researcher and leading academic authority on doctor-produced damage to mother and infant.

Do you want to know what can go wrong in hospital births—and what may have gone wrong with yours (even if you didn't recognize it)? *Birth Trap* will tell you—coolly, unemotionally, rationally, authoritatively, easily, and economically.

Do you want to know when—and how—to sue? Beginning with "Your selection of a lawyer is as important as the selection of your physician or midwife," Brackbill, Rice, and Young tell you, with case by case citations, comprehensively, in understandable English, not just *what* your legal rights are, but how you can begin to enforce them.

This volume is required reading for every law student and graduate lawyer in the field. Of course *Birth Trap* should be closely studied by doctors; but most of them will first discover it when they are hauled into court by their patients whose eyes have finally been opened.

Modern obstetrics will ultimately be destroyed not by the emotional and psychological benefits of home births but by public recognition of the real damage of hospital deliveries. Brackbill, Rice, and Young have fashioned the sword that every mother and father can use to counter the obstetrician's scalpel.

Read it yourself. Before you have a baby. After. Be sure your husband and your teen-age children read it. Use it for gifts to newlyweds. Or to grandparents who have been brainwashed into believing in hospital obstetrics. Send a copy to a medical student. Introduce your lawyer to it.

This book brings America a giant step closer to the time when no laboring mother will be allowed into a hospital without permission of a skilled midwife.

Robert S. Mendelsohn, M.D.

Author of *Malepractice: How Doctors Manipulate Women*
and *Confessions of a Medical Heretic*

Foreword

My hat is off to Yvonne Brackbill, June Rice, and Diony Young for their extraordinary book debunking the standard procedures in modern obstetrics, with hard statistical facts and cold logic, and at the same time including a strong overview of the existing state of the law showing your individual rights. The law will continue to change as the public, lawyers, judges, and, yes, doctors understand the problems caused by medical intervention. A fundamental in the law is that where there is a wrong there is a remedy. Unfortunately, sometimes it takes a very creative attorney to find the remedy to pierce the closed rank of the medical standard of practice.

Dr. Mendelsohn and the authors are correct in stating that your selection of an attorney is all important. Most lawyers are not engaged in litigation and still fewer have experience in the professional negligence arena. Nevertheless, most lawyers know how to find the specialist for you. After the lawyer specialist is selected, please do not be surprised if he or she advises not to sue. It may well be that although damage occurred, there is simply no standard in that community. Because of that, the doctor usually wins. However, if there has been an injury by all means explore the prospect of a suit. A large money judgment is another powerful tool by which to change harmful medical standards.

Be sure to take this book to your lawyer; it will be a valuable resource. It will help to evaluate the case as well as to pinpoint the necessary proof so that you may put together a winning effort.

Of course, the best "win" is not allowing the injury to happen in the first place.

All the money that a jury may award for an injured child is a poor substitute for a healthy child. And the best method to stop birth injuries by harmful intervention is to educate the public. I encourage every reader of this book to see that a copy is in every local library, but more importantly, in the hands of every mother-to-be.

Richard E. Hartman, *Esquire*

*Member of the Denver Bar, Member of the Colorado Bar,
Member of the American Bar, and Member of the American
Trial Lawyer's Association*

INTRODUCTION
High-Tech Birth Arrives

American families are changing in many ways. One important change is family size. In the days of our grandparents, large families were the rule. Today, large families are the exception. Most couples want only two children. In consequence, they are even more concerned that each child be normal and healthy.

Most babies will be normal and healthy if nothing goes wrong with their deliveries. However, because of the *technological* * *interventions* used in hospital obstetrics nowadays, many things can go wrong. Prospective parents need to be aware of these just as much as they need to read the fine print on any financial contract before signing it.

Another way in which families have changed is their appreciation of the birth experience. If you were born in the 1950s or early 1960s, chances are you were born in a hospital. Chances are also that neither of your parents was really present at your birth. Your father was not allowed to be present physically, and your mother, drugged to unconsciousness, was not present psychologically. When she awoke, she was in her room and you were in the nursery, separated from her and from your father by glass, an army of protective nurses, and a rigidly enforced 4-hour feeding schedule.

Nowadays, things are changing. Word is getting around that birthing is one of life's greatest experiences for parents as well as for baby.

*See Appendix A (Glossary) for the definition of this and other italicized terms.

Some medical practices are responding to these expectations. Yet some consumers believe that medical response is not enough, so that more and more parents are choosing to have their babies in a *free-standing birth center* or at home with a midwife. Still, the large majority of women choose in-hospital, rather than out-of-hospital, delivery on the assumption that in-hospital delivery minimizes physical risk.

But does it? In-hospital births, unlike out-of-hospital births, are high-technology deliveries, characterized by so-called interventions—timed labor, electronic fetal monitoring, ultrasound, drugs, and so on. Interventions are invasive procedures that literally interfere with the normal process of birth. That's why one obstetrician has called modern hospital obstetrics "meddlesome midwifery" and the modern obstetrician, an "intruder."

Presumably, every intervention was introduced into the technology of hospital birth because it was beneficial in some way to mother, infant, or hospital staff and because its benefits exceeded its risks. But people and circumstances change, and so do benefit/risk ratios. Also, some interventions have slipped into use without a proper evaluation in the first place. It is vitally important that all interventions be calculated periodically to ensure that their benefits exceed their risks. It is just as important that you, as prospective parents, have this information so that you can make your own informed decisions about choice of birth place, birth attendants, and the acceptability of interventions.

Chapter 1 of this book describes the most frequently used hospital interventions as well as their benefits and risks to mother and infant. Chapter 2 describes why hospitals and obstetricians find interventions beneficial. Chapter 3 discusses free-standing birth centers as an alternative to hospital or home delivery. In Chapter 4 out-of-hospital (low-tech) birthing is compared to in-hospital delivery. Chapter 5 invites you to make your own benefit/risk decision about accepting interventions and provides information needed to make such decisions.

Chapter 6 includes a discussion of various legal aspects to childbirth, such as obligations to the unborn child; the legal obligations of midwives, physicians, and hospital or clinic personnel; and a description of several types of legal suits used when childbirth does not result in a healthy, normal child, due to negligence on the part of physicians or others involved in childbirth. Chapter 7 discusses ways in which you, the consumer, can bring about changes in maternity care. In addition to facts, we have also included in all these chapters letters and comments from mothers about their own experiences.

Many people assume that their interests are being protected by their physicians or government regulatory agencies. This is simply not the case, as experience has shown. The foremost goal of this book is to impress upon you the need to be informed of both scientific and legal ramifications of technical childbirth so that you can best protect your rights and health, as well as those of your unborn child.

Contents

Birth Trap

THE LEGAL LOW-DOWN ON HIGH-TECH OBSTETRICS

1

High-Tech Interventions: Benefits and Risks of In-Hospital Delivery

For a variety of reasons (which will be discussed in Chapter 2), American medicine in general and hospital *obstetrics* in particular have always considered interventionism as their therapeutic model. Instead of letting nature take its course, American *obstetricians* take over.

Some of the most popular early interventions included the following. In the nineteenth century, bloodletting was fashionable therapy; the obstetrician accomplished it by puncturing a vein or by applying leeches to the woman's abdomen or *vagina* to suck out blood and thereby "relieve" localized aches and pains. Obstetricians often gave a purgative of calomel for puerperal fever, which might be followed by opium to counteract too large a dose of calomel. They gave emetics for convulsions, ergot to induce labor, and so on.[1] In the twentieth century, American obstetricians had their patients' vaginas douched with bichloride of mercury (now known to be a *teratogen*) and their heads shampooed with kerosene, ether, or ammonia.[1] Small wonder that the White House Conference on Child Health and Protection in its 1933 report entitled, "Fetal, newborn, and maternal mortality and morbidity," concluded that excessive intervention was a principal reason for excessive *maternal* and *infant mortality*.[1]

Today, the number of obstetrical interventions has increased rather than decreased. Chances of surviving a high-tech birth are better, but the more subtle risks are present in force and pervade every area: physical, psychological, emotional, and financial.

This chapter describes interventions that hospitals most frequently use in birthing, as well as the benefits and risks of those interventions. The sequence of descriptions follows the sequence in which, if you choose hospital birth, you are likely to encounter these instances of high technology, beginning with hospitalization itself.

Hospitalization

It is commonly assumed that it is safer to give birth in-hospital than out-of-hospital, but that assumption is being questioned because an increasing amount of research documents the risks of giving birth in-hospital (Chapter 2). At this point, however, we need to ask whether some hospitals are safer than others. According to a study by the *American College of Obstetricians and Gynecologists* (ACOG),[2] both infant and maternal death rates are highest for large hospitals with large obstetrical units (2000 or more births per year). They are also high in medical school hospitals and teaching hospitals affiliated with medical schools. Some of these deaths may reflect the greater number of high-risk mothers in large teaching hospitals. However,

> It is also likely that the greater tendency to intervene in the normal progress of labor and birth in these institutions, especially in order to provide learning opportunities for students and residents, contributes to the poorer maternal and infant outcome in these institutions and they also result in a disproportionately high incidence of neurologically damaged children.[3]

Mortality is not the only risk that differs among hospitals. *Morbidity* varies as well, particularly rates of hospital-originated infections. For some hospitals, infection rates following *cesarean sections* run as high as 50%.[4] Cesarean section rates also vary among hospitals. In the state of New York, for example, cesarean section rates for different hospitals vary from less than 1% to more than 25%.[5] This variation in rate is partly a result of hospital "aggressiveness" in policy regarding cesarean delivery and partly because of hospital size and teaching status. Large hospitals in which students learn how to do cesarean sections have a rate 50% higher than small hospitals.[6]

There are fewer scientific studies of the psychological risks of hospitalization than there are of the physical risks. Nevertheless, the major psychological risks can be inferred from the most frequent complaints of women about giving birth in hospitals. These complaints generally center around a set of negative emotions that *are* experienced (anxiety and fear, anger and resentment, depression and guilt) and a set of positive emotions that *may not* be experienced (love, attachment, joy, satisfaction, happiness). The emotions stem from the following circumstances surrounding hospitalization.

1. Loss of autonomy. Mothers find they have unwillingly relinquished control over themselves and over their own babies. "In the home, the baby belongs to the mother; in the hospital the baby belongs to the staff."[7] Mothers find themselves powerless and often unwillingly subject to interventions that they do not want and may believe to be harmful.

2. Loss of self-esteem. The hospitalized mother loses status as the center of attention shifts abruptly from her to the physician. "In the home, mother is queen bee; in the hospital, she is a transient boarder, lowest on the totem pole."[7]

3. Dehumanizing experiences and surroundings. The mother entering a hospital shares some experiences with the convict entering prison. Her own clothes and effects are removed. She dons a hospital-issued gown. The admissions clerk puts a hospital identification bracelet on her wrist, and that wrist may be fastened to the delivery table later. In teaching hospitals, she is the object of frequent *vaginal examinations* by staff and students who often fail to ask permission or even to introduce themselves. The hospitalized mother finds herself regarded as "*parturient* patient material" rather than as a human being. "Women are herded like sheep through an obstetrical assembly line. . . . Obstetricians today are businessmen who run baby factories."[1]

4. Exposure to unfamiliar surroundings and unfamiliar people. The hospitalized mother finds herself in the paradoxical situation of having to do something very intimate and very personal (giving birth) in a surrounding totally devoid of intimacy and in the company of totally unfamiliar people. The only person the mother knows — her obstetrician — typically does not arrive until a few minutes before delivery, if at all.

5. Frequent loss of critical opportunity to bond to the baby and to revitalize and strengthen existing bonds of love and attachment to the father. This loss is a consequence of such practices as separating father from mother at some point during delivery

(particularly when a cesarean delivery is done), using drugs that stupefy both mother and baby, and separating mother from baby following birth.

There are also economic risks in hospital delivery unless one is fully covered by health insurance. Hospitals charge for every item in every room the patient occupies, however briefly. Some hospitals charge for items that the patient may not use, for example, the services of an anesthesiologist when *anesthesia* is omitted. In 1981, the average cost of an uncomplicated delivery was $1600 in hospital charges and $639 in physician's fees, or $2239 total.[8] If the delivery is complicated, for example, by cesarean section, the total cost may be more than $7500.[8] In contrast, the average amount charged by a midwife for prenatal care, birth at home, and postnatal care is between $150 and $300.

Given this state of affairs, how did hospital births become so popular? Historically, the increase in hospital births coincided with physicians' successful takeover of obstetrics from *midwives* during the first part of this century. Efficiency is an all-pervasive criterion in medicine, and it is not efficient to spend time traveling to the homes of individual patients and then sitting for hours "watching a hole." Nor is it possible in this situation to increase income, teach large groups of students, or do the research that is required for professional advancement. The only way to achieve these goals is to centralize patients.[1]

In short, the push for *hospital births* came from physicians rather than from patients. Most American mothers today have never experienced an out-of-hospital birth and so have no basis for comparison. Reports from England, however, indicate that 86% of mothers who have experienced both choose *home births*, 10% choose hospital, and 4% have no preference. Those who prefer hospital birth tend to be poorer women whose own homes are crowded and who have no homemaker help during confinement.[9]

Shaving

Shaving the *perineal* area is routine in American hospitals. When asked why, physicians reply, "to avoid infection, since hair cannot be sterilized." The value of shaving is a belief unsupported by evidence, however. No scientific study has shown that shaving reduces rate of infection.[10,11] On the contrary, if there are any lacerations or abrasions produced by the razor, the risk of infection increases.

For most women, the major risk of shaving is not infection or even the itching and irritation caused when the hair begins to grow back. Far more important, according to mothers' complaints, are the psychological drawbacks. It is an unpleasant experience and one that contributes to feelings of dehumanization and loss of self-esteem. Shaving is also ". . . disturbing to the woman's feelings about her sexual attractiveness, already weakened after childbirth."[12]

Enemas

Giving enemas to women in labor is also routine and, like shaving, without scientific basis. Sometimes, in pushing the baby out, mothers push out *fecal matter* as well. Although esthetics and possible embarrassment may be legitimate concerns, enemas are not risk free. Enemas are unpleasant and uncomfortable. The increased *intraabdominal* pressure they generate tends to accelerate labor and make contractions harder to control. Enemas also may produce an imbalance of electrolytes (compounds in the blood), predisposing the mother to fatigue and other problems.[13] Nor do enemas reduce the incidence of contamination or infection.[14,15] Finally, the past association of enemas with illness may suggest to the mother that labor and delivery are unhealthy and sick, rather than normal functions.

Fasting

To labor is literally to work hard, and hard work requires energy from food. No one would think of asking a marathon runner to run on an empty stomach. Likewise, in most countries, no one expects a mother to starve while she labors to push out a baby. In American hospitals, however, laboring mothers are not allowed food and water. This schedule of deprivation, together with enemas, leaves mothers in a weakened condition and less able to cope successfully with the exertion of labor and delivery.

Why is something so contrary to common sense so common in America? American physicians' rationale is: Should *general anesthesia* be needed, stomach contents can be suctioned out. Note that the American rationale brings the *low-risk* client one step closer to becoming a *high-risk* patient by removing in advance an obstacle to intervention.

Intravenous Feeding (IVs)

In an attempt to compensate for depriving the mother of food and water, hospital personnel routinely insert a tube into a vein in the mother's arm through which fluid is administered. Although the mother receives some calories from the *dextrose* content of this *intravenous* fluid, the nutritional quality of that fluid is insufficient and inappropriate to her needs.

> Intravenous fluid ... guarantees negative nitrogen balance. Nitrogen balance is a condition of the body when the nitrogen taken in via the diet is equal to the nitrogen lost via the urine and feces. This is interpreted to mean that the person is adequately replacing the protein used up every day. But a woman in labor who is receiving intravenous fluids (which almost never contain protein) is not in nitrogen balance. This is because she continues to expend her body's store of protein, but it is not being replaced by the diet. This is a negative nitrogen balance—a condition of starvation.[13]

In addition, puncturing the skin's protective layers increases chances of a hospital-produced infection. Such infections

> are particularly dangerous for two reasons. First, they involve organisms that can survive in a hospital environment and that have become immune to standard treatment. Second, mother and child have never been exposed to this danger before and therefore have not established defense to the infection. The result is a greater chance of infection in the hospital that is more difficult to eradicate.[13]

IVs also impose another risk of quite a different order. When an IV needle is inserted into the mother's vein, it means that she is attached by a tube to a heavy bottle. This arrangement in effect immobilizes her. She cannot walk or exercise freely without pulling the needle out of her arm. Immobility has adverse consequences in and of itself: increases in length of labor, resorting to painkillers, use of *oxytocin*, and occurrence of fetal heart rate abnormalities.[16]

Induction

Hospitals emphasize speed and efficiency. Hospital space is limited and expensive. Every hospital service has its break-even point below which the service loses money, at which it pays for itself, and above which it makes a profit. Obstetrics is no exception. Delivery suites must reflect a high turnover rate to pay the mortgage on the first of the month and staff salaries every other Friday. From an economic point of view, hospitals cannot afford to allow women to labor at their own natural, unhurried pace. As one mother put it, "At [the hospital] people just wanted to hurry up and go home."[17]

In addition to speed and efficiency, hospital staff emphasize convenience. Like you, doctors and nurses prefer sleeping to working during late night hours. Patients are supposed to be sleeping then, too, and in this expectation, hospitals reduce night staff to skeleton crews. The pregnant reader can understand, then, that any intervention allowing labor to be speeded up as well as timed so that the baby will arrive between 8 AM and 4 PM Monday, Tuesday, Wednesday, Thursday, or Friday is not only highly valued by hospital administration and staff, but tends to become a routine, if not required, aspect of hospital delivery procedure.[18] (Obstetricians who attempt to manipulate birth to occur during normal working hours refer to this practice as "daylight obstetrics.")

Aside from the issue of convenience, are there medical *indications* (that is, reasons) for *induction* of labor? Broadly speaking, when the physician decides that the risks to the *fetus* of remaining in the *uterus* outweigh the risks of extrauterine existence, even as a *premature*, then he or she decides to terminate that *intrauterine* existence artificially by induction or by cesarean delivery. Intrauterine risks that may tip the balance in this decision include *Rh isoimmunization*, diabetes, *preeclampsia*, high blood pressure, kidney disease, and growth retardation. An occurrence that is not properly called a "risk" but that usually triggers the decision to induce is "postmaturity," that is, *gestational age* greater than 40 weeks.

Whether for convenience or medical indication, induction rates vary widely among hospitals, physicians, and time periods. For example, induction rates in hospitals in the United Kingdom vary from 15% to 55%.[19] In the early 1970s, some hospitals showed a marked increase in induction rates while other hospitals decreased their rates.[19] In the United States, the rate for whites was twice that for blacks.[20]

On the theoretical level, this "chaotic" variation suggests to statistical surveyors that induction rates are determined by opinion, convenience, and economics rather than the outcome of scientific studies. "One is . . . left wondering how a profession which has always thought of itself as scientific could have remained complacent in the face of such haphazard changes in practice."[19]

On the practical level, the pregnant consumer is well advised to inquire about the induction rate and policy of her potential obstetrician and of the hospital he or she uses. If the induction rate is low, she should also inquire about the cesarean section rate, since that is the alternative procedure for controlling childbirth by the criteria of convenience and efficiency.

Obstetricians induce labor by drugs or by *amniotomy*, surgically lacerating the protective membrane that holds the *amniotic fluid*. (This is also known as breaking the *bag of waters*.) The drug most commonly used to induce labor is oxytocin.[21] Oxytocin acts by stimulating the *uterine* muscle to contract. It is also used to augment or speed up labor.

Probably the chief risk of induction to the mother is the pain stemming from either method. Cutting into the *amnion* is painful, particularly if the *cervix* is not quite "ripe."[22] The contractions produced by oxytocin or any other uterine stimulant are unlike those produced naturally. Drug-produced contractions begin suddenly, recur more often, and are stronger than natural contractions. As one experienced mother said, "They grab instead of ripple." Most women find them difficult to bear without resort to painkillers. According to British figures, 50% of noninduced mothers make it through delivery without narcotics or other painkillers, but only 8% of induced mothers finish without resort to drugs.[23] In the extreme case, uterine muscle spasm or even rupture may occur.[19] Infection is another risk in those 20% to 30% of cases in which labor fails to begin soon after amniotomy. Induction also increases the probability that other interventions will follow, with attendant risks of their own. These interventions include fetal heart rate monitoring, anesthesia, forceps delivery, and cesarean section.[24]

Induction involves more risks for the baby than for the mother. Among the most serious is the risk of delivering a child not yet ready to be delivered—the risk of prematurity.[25] Associated with the risk of prematurity are risks of infant *respiratory distress syndrome*, a condition associated with immature lung development, increased length of hospitalization, developmental defects, and so on. Why is it difficult to be sure that a fetus is mature enough to leave the *womb*? Menstrual history is not always a valid index of gestational age, particularly for those women who have irregular menstrual periods or who have been taking *oral contraceptives*. There are newer ways of establishing fetal age, principally determining the *L/S ratio* from a sample of amniotic fluid and taking an *ultrasonographic* "picture" of the fetus, but neither is perfectly accurate nor known to be perfectly safe.

Another set of risks for the baby stems from loss of the amniotic fluid that protects the head and umbilical cord from excessive and uneven pressure during contractions. Without this fluid cushion, the baby's head becomes an unprotected battering ram as it moves down the birth canal, which increases the risk of misalignment of the cranial bones and intracranial hemorrhage, which may be accompanied by abnormal electroencephalogram (EEG) tracings.[26]

Interference with the oxygen supply to the baby is an ever-present risk from any method of induction. It may occur because of extremely strong contractions produced by oxytocin or, in the case of amniotomy, through compression of the umbilical cord. As less oxygen is delivered to the baby, its heart rate decreases and fetal distress may follow. Acidosis is a frequent consequence of induction, as is neonatal jaundice. Other types of infant morbidity have been documented.[19,22,27-32]

Electronic Fetal Monitoring

Hospitalized patients who are in labor now routinely undergo electronic fetal monitoring. The nurse places electrodes on the mother's abdomen and wraps a belt around her to hold them on ("indirect method") or else threads the wire through the vagina, through the cervix, and into the uterus, where the electrode is attached to the baby's scalp (the "direct method," requiring amniotomy). The fetal heartbeat is conveyed to the machine where it is displayed in analog form on an oscilloscope screen and is also printed out in digital form on paper tape. When the direct method is used, another needle is often inserted into the baby's head so that blood can be collected and analyzed for oxygen content.

Until recently, nurses and doctors monitored a baby's progress during birth by listening to the baby's heartbeat through a stethoscope placed on the mother's abdomen. In the 1950s, a physician invented a machine to do this monitoring electronically. During the 1960s, the electronic fetal monitor was refined and patented and started to roll off assembly lines. By the 1970s, it had become big business. "A system capable of both kinds of monitoring typically costs a hospital $6500 to $7500, depending on its sophistication, and adds $75 to $100 to the cost of a delivery. Six U.S. companies are in the business, with sales said to be running $25 to $30 million a year."[33]

At present, many delivery suites are well stocked with these expensive gadgets. To pay for them, hospitals routinize or even require their use. Some hospitals refuse admission to obstetrical patients who refuse electronic monitors, maintaining that "there is no such thing as a 'normal' labor," so that every woman should be monitored.[34] Obstetricians defend their use on the grounds that electronic monitors have reduced perinatal mortality. Is this true?

Infant and *perinatal mortality* have fallen during the 1970s. Manufacturers and other proponents of electronic monitoring attribute the fall in mortality to the rise in electronic monitoring. Critics argue that the concordance is coincidental and that the decrease in mortality is really attributable to a decrease in the number of unwanted pregnancies (through improved contraception and legalized *abortion*), to improved intrauterine environment for the fetus (through improved prenatal care, improved prenatal nutrition, and increased intervals between births), and to a decrease in the number of severely premature infants. Moreover, they point out, since electronic monitoring leads to a higher cesarean section rate (discussed below) and since the infant death rate attributable to cesarean delivery is double that for vaginal delivery, electronic fetal monitoring must lead to *higher* infant death rates rather than to *lower* death rates.

Critics also point out that despite all the published material devoted to electronic monitoring, only four methodologically sound studies have been carried out to evaluate this intervention.[35,36] In these studies, women in labor were randomly assigned to manually monitored and electronically monitored groups. The two groups of women were comparable in other respects. Results were the same in all four studies: more electronically monitored women ended up in the operating room with cesarean deliveries. Cesarean section rates ranged between 63% and 314% higher for electronically monitored women than manually monitored women. There was no improvement in perinatal outcome for the babies delivered by cesarean section. The principal "reasons" alleged for these surgical deliveries—fetal distress and *cephalopelvic disproportion* (disproportion of head to pelvis)—cannot be proved or disproved. The real reasons, according to these studies, are attending physicians' impatience and nervousness.[37,38]

Problems of scientific soundness aside, no research is required to document many of the drawbacks and risks associated with use of electronic monitoring by either internal or external methods. Both methods have risks in common. One risk is that the mother is immobilized and recumbent. Not being able to move about lowers blood pressure, which in turn decreases the oxygen supply to the fetus, which in turn produces abnormalities in heart rate. Therefore, electronic monitoring tends to produce the very abnormalities it is supposed to measure. Other risks shared by both methods include the unknown risk of ultrasound, when this is part of the monitoring, and that of keeping alive a severely handicapped infant who might otherwise have died.[39]

Internal monitoring exposes both mother and baby to serious risks. One such risk is maternal infection from puncturing the amnion and introducing electrodes into her body. "This in-dwelling equipment provides a possible route for the entry of bacteria from the vagina and endocervix into the amniotic fluid.[40] Infection rate in internally monitored women is double that of manually monitored women.[41] Cultures of amniotic fluid taken during electronic monitoring show potentially dangerous bacteria in 50% of monitored women. The risk of infection increases the longer internal monitoring continues.[39] When monitoring continues more than 4½ hours, the risk of infection is 50%.[42] If it were not for antibiotics, the death rate from monitor-produced infection would be staggering. On the other hand, one should not forget that the use of antibiotics ". . . places the mother at risk of antibiotic side effects, fosters the growth of resistant organisms, and complicates care of the newborn."[35] The baby is also at risk of infection from the scalp-implanted internal electrodes. For example, several cases of herpes simplex have been transmitted by this method of fetal monitoring.[43]

In internal monitoring, the electrodes themselves frequently lacerate the cervix, vagina, and rectum while they are being inserted, thus increasing the risk of infection and hemorrhage. Puncturing the uterus has also been reported. The mother is not the only electrode victim, of course. Of all internally monitored babies, 4% to 5% suffer scalp abscesses, scalp lacerations, hematomas, and hemorrhages. Leakage of cerebrospinal fluid has also been recorded. Because amniotomy must be done before electrodes can be inserted, there is a sharp increase in the risk of prolapsed cord and resulting fetal distress. Here again, note that electronic monitoring is producing the risk it is supposed to measure. (Many mothers leave the hospital firmly convinced that electronic monitoring saved their babies from otherwise certain death caused by cord prolapse when in fact it was the monitoring [and prerequisite amniotomy] that caused the prolapse in the first place.)

When the external method of monitoring is used, the patient stands a lower chance of infection and trauma but a higher chance of being rushed to the operating room because of measurement errors. As experts explain it,

> All of the external techniques for recording fetal heart rate data use electronic logic; because of this electronic logic, fetal heart rate data are not identical to ECG beat-to-beat heart rate. The most significant problem related to the ultrasonic fetal heart rate record is the artifactually introduced, apparently increased baseline fetal heart rate variability. This may lead to a false sense of normal variability when, in reality, the baseline is smooth. In addition, subtle periodic changes may be obscured. Another problem with ultrasound instrumentation is that the fetal heart rate may double at low rates and can be halved at high rates.[42]

It is also possible to confuse maternal heart rate with fetal heart rate.

> The maternal electrocardiogram has been recorded instead of the fetal heart rate in patients with fetal death. Maternal and fetal heart rate have been added together, producing a spurious *tachycardia* (rapid heart rate), and totally spurious results have been recorded.[40]

The bottom line is that the external method of monitoring is plagued by measurement artifacts that lead to misinterpretation of normal stress for fetal distress and vice versa.

Horizontal (Supine, Lithotomy) Position

Trying to birth a baby while lying flat on a table is unnatural and very difficult. As one obstetrician said, "Except for being hanged by the feet, the supine position is the worst conceivable position for labor and delivery."[44] Another physician writes, "No other animal species adopts such a disadvantageous posture during such an important and critical event."[45]

When given a free choice, 95% of women prefer some position in which labor and gravity are in phase: they sit, kneel, squat, stand, or walk about during labor, varying their position according to the dictates of comfort and the position of the child's head in the pelvis.[46] Why, then, do most hospitalized women end up flat on their backs, with their hands immobilized and their legs up in the air?

Many obstetricians prefer the *lithotomy position* because they do not have to squat or bend down. They also like it because it facilitates intervention procedures, for example, *episiotomy* and extracting the baby with *forceps*. Another reason suggested for the popularity of the horizontal position is that this position helps some obstetricians remove the last vestige of self-esteem from the mother. "When the mother is lying down, it's the doctor who is having the baby. When the mother is sitting up, it is she who's having it. Many doctors don't like that."[47]

Does the mother's position make any difference? It makes many differences, none in favor of the *supine position*. First, the horizontal position increases the length of labor.[48] In addition, the heavy uterus compresses major blood vessels, interfering with circulation and decreasing blood pressure,[49-51] which in turn lowers oxygen supply to the fetus and increases the risk of fetal distress and *asphyxia*.[16,51] The immobility and compression are uncomfortable, increasing the need for painkillers.[16,52] The horizontal position also increases the need for episiotomy because of disproportionate tension on the *pelvic floor* and stretching of the perineal tissue.[53] Because the baby's passage through the birth canal must work against gravity when the mother is supine, cephalopelvic disproportion is more frequently diagnosed (a frequent consequence of which is a cesarean section),[40] forceps extraction is more frequently required,[48] and physical injuries to the baby are more numerous.[54] Finally, many mothers report that their labor is slowed because of their fear that the baby will fall over the edge of the table with no one there to catch it.

Vaginal Examinations

After the electronic fetal monitor is attached to the mother, the nurse repeatedly checks it. So do other medical personnel and students.[55] Numerous hands explore the mother's vagina—adjusting equipment, testing to see if everything is in order. Chances are that one of these hands will introduce a microorganism that will find one small vaginal laceration and produce a serious infection.

In a study[56] comparing deliveries monitored with and without electronic devices, researchers found the postpartum infection rate to be significantly higher among electronically monitored patients, a difference that probably reflects the excessive number of vaginal examinations for the electronically monitored group. One mother recounts her personal experience in this respect,

> Typically they'd come in and say to make frog legs. Then they'd stick their finger up me and leave. Well, one of those times turned out to be an artificial rupture. I found out about that a couple of hours later.[17]

Thanks to *antibiotics*, infections no longer pose a major threat to life itself. Nevertheless, antibiotics themselves carry minor risks for mothers and are a major problem for breast-fed babies, since they are excreted in breast milk.

Quite apart from electronic fetal monitoring, excessive vaginal exams are a frequent complaint of women who deliver in university-affiliated or teaching hospitals, that is, hospitals accommodating students, interns, and residents. All these young apprentices need to practice on real people and, like it or not, their practice material includes you. As one mother put it, "I reached the point where I wouldn't have been surprised if the man who was washing the windows had suddenly laid down the sponge and come over to 'take a peek.' It seemed that everyone connected with the hospital was doing it."[1] The future holds little promise for correction of this problem. At a recent meeting of the Central Association of Obstetricians and Gynecologists, it was strongly recommended that vaginal exams be carried out routinely, every hour.[57]

Episiotomy

Episiotomy is a surgical operation in which the skin around the vaginal opening (the *perineum*) is cut to enlarge the opening for birth. Following birth, the cut must be sewn up and the vaginal opening reconstructed.

Why an episiotomy? U.S. physicians allege the major benefit of this operation is to forestall future flabbiness in the perineum ("pelvic floor incompetence" or "*pelvic relaxation*"). Strangely enough, however, there are no hard facts to support this contention. According to one group of researchers,

> Episiotomy has been the norm in American obstetrics since about 1930. One of the rationales for this has been the widespread belief among physicians that doing an episiotomy protects against later pelvic relaxation and prevents the need for corrective surgery later in life. We could find no scientific justification for this in the literature although in 1920 it appeared in *Williams' Obstetrics* textbook stated as a belief and has been there ever since. By the 1975 edition of *Williams' Obstetrics* it is stated as fact.[58]

Long-term, follow-up data from the Netherlands[59] and the United States[58] indicate that there is no cause-effect relationship between episiotomy and pelvic relaxation. The incidence of pelvic relaxation has been declining in both countries, independent of episiotomy rates. The same conclusion emerges from comparing data for Scandinavia, where the episiotomy rate is 3%, with data from the United States and England, where episiotomy for primigravidas is routine in many hospitals.[60]

A second reason for episiotomy, advanced by U.S. obstetricians, is to avoid tearing the perineum as the baby's head emerges. Here again, there are no data to support this rationale. Quite the contrary, vaginal deliveries in-hospital yield a significantly higher rate of perineal lacerations than do out-of-hospital deliveries, despite the fact that episiotomies routinely accompany hospital deliveries. One American study found nine times as many severe tears in hospital deliveries as in home births, even though there were also nine times as many episiotomies among the hospital deliveries.[54] An English study found that despite a two-fold increase in episiotomies at one major hospital, the number of perineal tears did not decline.[61]

A third rationale favoring episiotomy, according to some obstetricians, is that it speeds up the second stage of labor, thereby shortening the time during which the baby's head is under pressure, which in turn reduces the probability of brain damage. However, studies tracing the causes of mental and motor abnormalities in infants find no significant associations between these abnormalities and the length of the second stage of labor.[62] On the contrary, most interventions applied for the purpose of speeding labor (for example, use of amniotomy, oxytocin, forceps) are associated with risks for both mother and baby.

If the benefits of episiotomy are questionable, what about the risks? No question here; there are risks for both the mother and the baby. For the mother, several risks are connected with the surgery itself. First, there is a risk that the obstetrician will cut the nerve supply to the anus. A second risk is that in sewing up the incision, the obstetrician will reconstruct the vaginal opening so that it is too small or too large for sexual compatibility. There is also a risk that the wound will become infected postoperatively. (Death from such infections accounted for 20% of all maternal mortality in King County, Washington and 5% of all maternal mortality in the entire state between 1969 and 1977.)[63]

The most frequently encountered risk from episiotomy is the pain it produces—pain likely to be more intense and longer lasting than that resulting from a naturally occurring tear. Feelings of pain, general discomfort, or numbness may persist for months or years. Some women experience the pain only during intercourse, which tends to interfere with sexual pleasure and orgasm.[64] As one noninterventionist physician commented,

> Very few mothers are aware of the possibility that a fourth-degree episiotomy is becoming more and more common in an effort to "save the baby"—although in this case it is at the expense of the mother's short-term comfort and possibly her long-term functioning as well. Also, whereas the pains involved in giving birth are meaningful, the pain afterward from stitches or a rectal or anal wound is not meaningful.[65]

For the baby, drug effects are the major risks of episiotomy. Since the surgery and repair are painful, the mother is generally given an anesthetic agent. Predelivery anesthetic agents reach the baby within a few minutes of administration. Postdelivery anesthetic agents reach breastfed babies because they are excreted in breast milk. Withholding an anesthetic when the mother wants it can also produce its own set of problems, as one upset mother recalls:

> I need medical advice because of the butchered episiotomy they gave me. It seems to *not* be healing and I'm scared! They *wouldn't* even give me a local while they did repairs. . . . I was treated so *terribly*—so inhumanely—that even after 2½ weeks now I have nightmares day and night. It's *awful*. I happened to pass the hospital the other day, and I just broke down.[66]

Obstetrical Drugs

Hospitals may withhold food to mothers who are in labor, but they treat them to a pharmaceutical feast. The enema she receives contains soapsuds. Dripping through the IV tube into her arm are dextrose and saline and, often, oxytocin *(Pitocin)* to start labor contractions or speed them up. She is offered *sedative-hypnotics* for fear and apprehension, *narcotics* for labor pains, tranquilizers to augment the narcotics, *amnesics* to obliterate the memory of pain, *narcotic antagonists* to reduce the adverse side effects of narcotics on the baby, *antiemetics* to reduce the adverse side effects of narcotics, anesthetics for pain of delivery, *vasoconstrictors* to reduce the adverse effects of the anesthetics, *antacids* to reduce the adverse effects of the anesthetics, and more oxytocin to hurry expulsion of the placenta or, in the case of cesarean sections, more narcotics for pain as well as *prophylactic* antibiotics to head off the high probability of infection.

The ultimate reason for administering most drugs in hospital birth is pain related. Nevertheless, relief from pain is not without cost to the mother. At the extreme of physiological risks is anesthetic-related death. Although death is not very common, adverse physiological reactions are. Painkillers slow labor or bring it to a stop altogether, which in turn requires oxytocin to "augment" labor, which in turn increases pain and the need for more painkillers. Painkillers also decrease maternal blood pressure, which reduces the oxygen supply to the fetus. An insufficient oxygen supply tends to trigger an abnormal heart rate, which places both mother and baby at risk for cesarean section. Administration of a regional anesthetic (for example, *epidural*) always interferes with blood pressure and is sometimes followed by severe headache, toxic reactions, and neurological impairment.

In addition to physiological adverse drug reactions, obstetrical drugs have adverse psychological effects for the mother. All anesthetic and preanesthetic medications decrease maternal alertness and thus may interfere with bonding. If the mother has had heavy medication, she will not be conscious at all when her baby is born. In addition, narcotic painkillers are often associated with *postpartum depression*.

For mothers, the benefits of obstetrical drugs for pain relief may outweigh their physiological and psychological risks. For babies, however, the case is different. The fetus is not in pain. It has no need of dextrose, saline, oxytocin, sedative-hypnotics, narcotics, tranquilizers, amnesics, antiemetics, vasoconstrictors, or anesthetics. These drugs do not benefit the baby. Instead, they pose substantial risks.

To appreciate the full extent of drug risks for babies, one must remember that brain development is not complete at time of birth. The brain continues to develop for at least 2 postnatal years, and during this period it is especially susceptible to injury.[67] Drugs, such as aspirin that adults can consume without a second thought may be toxic for an infant, causing small but permanent damage to its still developing central nervous system. All drugs used in obstetrics are toxic for infants. With few exceptions, obstetrical drugs cross the *placenta* and enter fetal circulation within a few minutes of their administration to the mother. Studies of babies whose mothers have received obstetrical drugs have repeatedly and consistently demonstrated the sort of adverse effects that are associated with central nervous system damage: impaired sensory and motor responses; reduced ability to process incoming stimuli and control responding to them; interference with feeding, sucking, and rooting responses; lower scores on tests of infant development; and increased irritability. *Bonding* may also be impaired.[68]

Obstetrical drugs also produce adverse physical and physiological effects in the baby. The most frequently occurring physiological changes include respiratory depression, general sluggishness and fatigue, extremes of muscular tone (limpness or rigidity), skin discoloration (blue instead of pink), increased *bilirubin* level and jaundice, abnormal EEG and sleep/alertness patterns, and increased tremulousness.[68,69]

How could it be possible that obstetric drugs produce so many adverse, harmful effects? Isn't the *Food and Drug Administration (FDA)* responsible for approving drugs on the basis of their safety and effectiveness? If the FDA has approved these drugs, how can they be unsafe?

Yes, the law requires that the FDA approve a drug as safe and effective before releasing it for clinical use. However, FDA approval is for certain specified and limited uses. For example, *ketamine*, a general anesthetic, was developed for use in certain diagnostic and surgical procedures not requiring skeletal muscle relaxation. The FDA approved it for those purposes. The FDA did not approve it for use in labor and delivery. In fact, the FDA requires the manufacturer to print the following warning on the ketamine package insert: "Since the safe use [of ketamine] in pregnancy, including obstetrics . . . has not been established, such use is not recommended." Nevertheless, ketamine is being used in labor and delivery. According to the FDA, its use in labor and delivery is not the FDA's responsibility. It is, instead, the physician's responsibility. The FDA simply regards it as an experimental drug when it is used for a nonapproved purpose.[70]

With few exceptions, the drugs most commonly used in childbirth are in the same situation. They have been approved by the FDA for use in other conditions. They have not been approved by the FDA for use in obstetrics. When they are used in obstetrics, they are legally "experimental" drugs and the FDA assumes no responsibility for their safety or effectiveness.[70]

Balancing Benefits Against Risks

Since obstetrical medication is chiefly pain related, one wants to know just how painful childbirth is. How many women could deliver without painkillers? Are drugs used in most hospital births? Does hospital delivery intensify pain?

Recent pharmacological research[71] indicates that the pain threshold increases during pregnancy and particularly during labor and delivery. In other words, given the same stimulus, women who are in labor feel less pain than women who are not in labor. Nevertheless, there are wide individual differences in the amount of pain that women report, probably reflecting differences in pain threshold, type and amount of prenatal training, physical factors in both the mother and the baby, and circumstances surrounding birth. Just before the end of the second stage of labor, many women delivering without drugs experience some discomfort. If they are tired and labor has been long, they are likely to feel that they "can't go on without something." This final stage, just before the baby's head emerges, normally lasts only a few minutes and is the point at which experienced midwives provide comforting words and acts rather than drugs. Once the cervix is fully dilated and the mother feels the urge to push, she may no longer experience pain, as long as she keeps pushing.

It is difficult to say how many women *could* deliver without painkillers because nearly all deliver in hospitals and nearly all deliver with drugs. Dr. Pierre Vellay, the French advocate of "painless labor," estimates, on the basis of some 40,000 deliveries, that 75% of women could deliver without anesthesia.[72] Kloosterman, of the Netherlands, estimates that 80% to 90% of women are capable of delivering without any intervention, including drugs.[45] For American women who deliver out-of-hospital, the estimated number delivering without anesthesia is closer to 100%. Dr. Robert Bradley, a Denver physician and author specializing in natural childbirth since the 1940s, has attended some 14,000 births and reports a 96.4% rate of completely drugless births. The Farm, a religious community in central Tennessee, has had 1200 births over 10 years and reports a rate of 98.1% without interventions, including no drugs and no devices.[73]

Are drugs used in most hospital births? Yes. Hospitalized obstetrical patients received 4.8 million doses of *analgesics*, 1.3 million doses of sedatives, and 1.1 million doses of tranquilizers in 1977.[74] Unaware of this, most women enter the hospital with the expectation that they will not have to take any drugs. Nevertheless, close to 100% receive at least one drug[75] and the majority, including *Lamaze*-trained mothers, receive many more than that.[75] One study reports an average of seven different drug administrations during vaginal delivery and 15.2 during cesarean delivery.[76] Worse yet, many of these drugs are documented teratogens or *toxins*. According to one study,[75] 86% of mothers who deliver in-hospital receive at least one teratogenic drug during childbirth and 64% receive at least two.[77] These percentages are even higher for mothers who deliver surgically.

Does hospital delivery intensify pain? Many factors associated with hospital delivery actually do increase pain, so that it is literally true that women who deliver in-hospital experience more pain. Of great significance here is the fact that most obstetrical interventions increase pain, either directly or indirectly, so that hospital delivery to a considerable extent creates its own market for painkillers. Intervention techniques that increase pain include enemas, supine position, electronic fetal monitoring, amniotomy, oxytocin, and cesarean section. The unreal, dehumanizing hospital atmosphere also contributes to pain. As one obstetrician has noted, "pain thrives on fear, on lack of confidence, and on loneliness."[45] All of these qualities characterize hospitals, and all act in psychological concert to intensify pain. In addition, nursing and medical staff reinforce the expectation of pain and hold out the promise, frequently in a very persuasive way, of drugs to relieve pain—even when the mother has not asked for drugs.

Why do obstetricians use drugs? Obstetricians rely on drugs for a variety of reasons. One is that drugs provide an easy way to maintain control over patients. Drugged patients are usually quiet, compliant, and easily manipulated. Another reason has to do with obstetricians justifying their presence (and their fees) in a situation that the mother and the nurse could probably manage successfully by themselves. Physicians are the only ones who can prescribe drugs, so by making it seem that drugs are indispensable, physicians also make it seem that they are indispensable. Additionally, some physicians reason that the mothers' relief from pain will make them feel grateful and indebted to their physicians.

Drugs not only increase power over patients but also power over time. They contribute enormously to predictability, routinization, and convenience of birth events.[78] For example, the use of oxytocin to precipitate or speed up labor allows uninterrupted nighttime sleep and free weekends. (An unexpectedly small number of babies are born on Saturdays, Sundays, and holidays.[18,79,80]) The use of narcotics to slow labor allows births to be postponed to a more convenient time. To the professional, time is of the essence; it is equivalent to money. Every minute saved from one patient can be invested profitably in some other pursuit or in adding another patient to the total case load.

A more obvious economic reason for using drugs in hospital births is that one professional specialty, obstetrical anesthesiology, exists solely for alleviating pain. If painkillers were to be deemphasized, the very reason for the existence of the jobs and salaries of many professionals would disappear.

Mechanical Extraction of the Baby

The forceps is an instrument used for pulling a baby out of the birth canal. It operates like a pair of tongs or pliers. On one end of the forceps are clamps that are inserted into the birth canal until they grasp the baby's head. The physician then squeezes the handles on the other end and pulls. The terms *low forceps, mid forceps,* and *high forceps* indicate how far the instrument is inserted into the birth canal.

The *vacuum extractor,* another instrument for removing the baby, works on a different principle. This instrument has a suction cup on the operative end that attaches to the infant's scalp and pulls the baby down and out of the birth canal. The operative principle is much like that underlying first trimester vacuum-assisted abortions. Physicians are most likely to use mechanical extraction when they decide that labor is not progressing fast enough.

In U.S. hospitals, *mechanical extraction* with forceps is used in 5% to 20% of deliveries.[54] Vacuum extraction is used in less than 5% of deliveries. The forceps delivery rate used to be much higher but has been supplanted in popularity by cesarean delivery, which accomplishes the same thing—prompt removal of the baby. In some European hospitals, for example, those in Sweden, mechanical extraction is still favored over cesarean. In other countries, for example, Israel,[81] mechanical extraction and cesarean delivery are used in combination.

Mechanical extraction is rarely used in home births. In a study of 2092 home and hospital births in which material participants were matched on age and parity, Mehl found forceps used in less than 1% of home deliveries. Hospital birth statistics presented a sharp contrast: mid forceps were used in 20% and low forceps in 11% of deliveries.[54]

Since the use of forceps is much higher in in-hospital than in out-of-hospital deliveries, does this suggest that *failure to progress* is more likely to occur in-hospital? Yes. There are many ways in which hospitals may inhibit labor. The use of drugs and the generation of fear are two examples. In addition, hospital emphasis on speed and efficiency leads medical personnel to call "slow" or "failing to progress" many labors that out-of-hospital birth attendants would call "within normal limits." In an English study, a first-time mother reported that the hospital nurse warned her ". . . that the second stage was not permitted to last longer than 30 minutes. The urge to push receded while I lay in terror."[82]

Mechanical extraction is risky for both mother and baby. For mother, having a good sized pair of tongs inserted into the vagina, through the cervix, and into the uterus is understandably painful and requires a painkilling drug, which in turn adds drug effects to the list of risks for the baby. Additionally, there is the risk of rupturing the mother's uterus as well as lacerating her vagina.

For the baby, the chief risk from the use of forceps is mechanically inflicted damage, including bruising; intracranial hemorrhage; hematoma (swelling filled with blood); bone deformation damage to facial and brachial nerves; and damage to eyes, spinal cord, and brain stem.[54] The perinatal death rate associated with use of forceps is 8 deaths per 10,000 births, according to a recent British study.[83]

Vacuum extraction is presumably less risky for babies than is forceps.[84] Nevertheless, all vacuum-extracted babies have, at the very minimum, a superficial scalp lesion where the rim of the suction cup attached to the scalp and pulled the head. Although most of these lesions heal within a few days, about 13%[85] are more serious and require treatment. Hematoma occurs in about 6% of vacuum-extracted babies[85] and requires several weeks to heal. Indications of neurological damage (for example, convulsions, spasticity, retinal hemorrhage, abnormal EEG) occur in 3.3% of vacuum-extracted babies.[85] The perinatal death rate associated with vacuum extraction is 15.5 deaths per 1000 extractions.[85]

Although vacuum extraction poses no physical risks to the mother, it does pose psychological risks. Following vacuum extraction, the baby's head is always unbeautiful, sometimes even "unsightly and alarming."[85] The baby's impaired physical appearance may well interfere with bonding; certainly, it does nothing to enhance attachment.

Cesarean Section

An alternative procedure for extracting the baby quickly is to cut into the mother's abdomen and take the baby out. This procedure, called cesarean section[86] or c-section, is major surgery. The most popular type is a "low" section, done by making a horizontal cut into the lower abdomen and uterus.

When do doctors decide to perform a cesarean section? The most common reason, or "indication" in medical jargon, is when a previous delivery was by cesarean section.[87] Apart from repeat sections, the most frequently cited reason is *dystocia* (prolonged labor). Other cited reasons include fetopelvic disproportion, fetal distress (determined by heart rate); unusual fetal positions, including breech; conditions associated with placental hemorrhage[88]; prolapse (falling down) of the umbilical cord; certain preexisting medical conditions such as diabetes, venereal disease, or toxemia; and prolonged or premature rupture of the membranes.[88]

Cesarean sections were rare events when most births took place at home. Homes are just not suitable places for carrying out major surgery. Consequently, for the first two decades of this century, the cesarean section rate was 1% to 3% for most parts of the U.S. Then, in the 1930s, as the hospital became the principal place of birth, surgical births began to increase. From the mid-1960s through the mid-1970s the surgical delivery rate increased each year by 12% to 20% — even in years when the birthrate itself was decreasing.[6] By 1982, the cesarean section rate for the country as a whole reached 18%,[89] and there are indications that the increase will continue.

Benefits and Risks of Cesarean Deliveries for Babies

What are the benefits and risks of surgical birth? Even obstetricians make no claim of benefits for mothers, maintaining instead that a cesarean delivery is a baby-oriented procedure. But is it? Do the risks of surgical birth outweigh its benefits? What are these risks?

The bottom line for risks is mortality, and that is four times higher for infants delivered surgically than for infants delivered vaginally.[90] Morbidity rates are also excessive for babies delivered surgically; their overall rate of illness is ten times higher than for vaginally delivered babies.[90] These illnesses have many sources. One stems from the fact that the intense pain of major surgery cannot be borne without recourse to analgesics and anesthetics. For this reason, cesarean deliveries require strong drugs and lots of them.[76,91] Consequently, babies born by cesarean section are automatically exposed to damage from the toxic and teratogenic compounds described earlier.

Since postoperative pain is also intense, powerful analgesics, typically narcotics, are also needed for several days. These drugs make their way into breast milk[92] just as easily as they cross the placenta. The consequences are the same for the baby in either case. The mother who has a cesarean birth and who wishes to breastfeed must either sanction this risk or postpone breastfeeding until she is drug free. Neither option is a good one for the baby.

Another major risk is that the obstetrician may operate before the fetus is ready to be delivered. About 6% to 7% of babies born through the normal, vaginal route are *premature* (or *preterm*). However, the prematurity rate for babies born by elective cesarean section is three times as high.[6] One consequence of prematurity is the increased risk that the baby's lungs will be too immature to deliver enough oxygen to the body. This condition is called *respiratory distress syndrome* (formerly, *hyaline membrane disease*). Death resulting from respiratory distress syndrome is seven times greater in premature infants delivered operatively than in those delivered vaginally.[93,94] Another consequence of prematurity is an increased probability that the baby will be sent to the intensive care unit (ICU) nursery, which has all the problems of the normal nursery and then some. About 30% of the babies prematurely delivered by cesarean section become candidates for intensive care because they are seriously ill.[6]

Another unavoidable risk is that surgically born babies remain in the hospital about three times longer than their normally born counterparts. This longer stay in the hospital increases their exposure to nursery-borne infections and diseases, triples their hospital bills, and decreases their chances of an early established strong bond with parents.

Finally, the more premature the infant, the greater the chances that it will be defective physically and mentally. One such outcome is cerebral palsy.[95] As one pediatrician recently noted, "Advances in newborn intensive care have dramatically increased the survival of very low-birth-weight infants, but survival for many infants has been blemished by visual impairment, including total blindness in some, developmental delay, or neurologic problems.[96]

So much for the risks from surgical birth. What are the alleged benefits for the baby? Physicians claim the benefit of a cesarean section is a "superior outcome" for baby.[6] When asked for documentation that cesarean deliveries produce a "high quality product," physicians point to a significant decline in perinatal and neonatal death rates for 1966 to 1975. Statisticians, however, caution that a relationship does not necessarily indicate a cause-effect relationship and point to the other changes occurring during that 10-year period that might have caused the decline in early mortality: increase in infant health-promoting services, such as well-baby clinics and immunizations; improvement in maternal diet and welfare-supported dietary supplements for poor mothers; and increased availability of *contraceptive* and abortion services. They also point to the fact that while the United States shot well ahead of all other countries in surgical deliveries, its relative order with respect to perinatal and infant mortality did not change. In 1974–1975, the death rate for full-term infants born vaginally was 12 deaths per 1000 live births; for full-term infants born surgically, the rate was 34 deaths per 1000 live births; and for preterm infants born surgically and weighing less than 1250 grams (about 2.75 lbs.), the death rate was 87 deaths per 1000 live births.[19]

Risks of Surgical Delivery for Mothers

As we pointed out earlier, physicians do not try to rationalize cesarean surgery in terms of physical benefits for mothers. There are no benefits for mothers. There are plenty of risks, however.

Mortality. Death is not the most common risk of cesarean section, but it is the most serious one. Maternal death rates are substantially higher during and after surgical delivery than vaginal delivery. In California, the death rate for cesarean sections is 2.4 times that of vaginal delivery. In Rhode Island, the death rate for cesarean sections is 26 times that of vaginal delivery.[6] A significant number of deaths in cesarean deliveries are from complications of anesthesia.[19]

Physiological risks. Infection following a cesarean birth is a high probability risk, occurring in up to half the mothers undergoing such surgery,[97] despite the widespread policy of administering prophylactic antibiotics to all mothers who have a surgical delivery. The most common types of infection are intrauterine cystitis (inflammation resulting from bacterial infection); peritonitis (inflammation of the membrane that lines the abdominal walls); abscess, gangrene, and sepsis (poisoning as a consequence of putrefaction); urinary tract infection; and respiratory infection.[35]

Hemorrhage is another common complication of surgical delivery. Transfusion follows cesarean section in 10% to 14% of all cases.[6]

Severe pain is an inevitable consequence of major surgery. Cesarean section is no exception. Operative administration of an anesthetic is a must, and postoperative administration of narcotic painkillers is routine. The risk for the baby—drugs passed across the placenta and excreted in breast milk—has already been pointed out. For the mother, the chief risk from consuming strong painkillers is probably the depression that follows the termination of their use. Narcotic-induced sleep and sluggishness may also interfere with mother-infant bonding. (Sluggishness and fatigue may last several weeks.)

Other side effects that have been encountered during or after surgical delivery include gas; adhesions; *fistula*; gaps or splitting of the
wound (wound "dehiscence"); uterine rupture; injury to adjacent organs, principally bladder and bowel; blood transfusion complications,
including hepatitis, incompatibilities, and coagulation; thromboemboli
(blocking of a blood vessel by a blood clot); thrombophlebitis (venous inflammation and clotting at the site); *aspiration pneumonia* and other accidents of anesthesia; cardiac arrest; and cerebral vascular accidents.[98]

Emotional and psychological risks. Most mothers who have cesarean births experience guilt, anger, depression, and feelings of helplessness following their surgery. Many blame themselves for failing ("if
I had just tried a little harder"). Others are angry and depressed because
they have been given no information about what is going on, have had
no role in the decision-making process, and have not played a real part
in the delivery. The depression is a long-lasting one,[99] particularly if the
mother has no supportive family member to help, nurture, and reassure
her.[100]

> In my own research, I observed that women who had been delivered by
> cesarean were significantly more negative about their birth experience,
> were much more miserable physically, required far more drugs postpar-
> tum, experienced more serious and longer lasting depression, and did not
> "feel like a mother" (a measure of attachment and bonding) till much later
> than the vaginally delivered women. Many other researchers have re-
> ported on the shock, deep disappointment, feelings of failure and other
> negative emotions experienced by cesarean mothers postpartum. Surgery
> is never a pleasant experience, but becoming a mother through major ab-
> dominal surgery is particularly difficult. Helpless dependent newborns
> cannot wait until their mothers "recover"—they need mothering at
> once.[101]

Unfortunately, hospitals' and physicians' resistance to allowing
support is even greater than the mother's need for support. Parents' biggest wish is to remain together during delivery, but most operating
rooms are off limits to fathers and advocate-companions. Obstetricians,
and particularly obstetrical anesthesiologists, rationalize their closed
door policy by claiming that a maternal companion would take up too
much space, introduce infection, become ill or faint, interfere with the
operation, or bring a lawsuit.[6] (None of these claims has been documented.) The result is that mothers are separated from loved ones and
from their babies, and these separations intensify negative experiences
and emotions.

Not the least of the psychological costs of cesarean deliveries is the anticipation of future cesarean sections for subsequent pregnancies. U.S. obstetricians, worried by the prospect of uterine rupture and malpractice suits, follow the dictum "once a cesarean, always a cesarean."[102] Thus 99% of American women who have delivered once by cesarean section are forced to deliver again by cesarean section. In many other countries, obstetricians allow their patients to have a "trial of labor," since the probability of uterine rupture is very low[103] and the probability of success is very high if the reason for the first surgical delivery is nonrecurring. In fact, in one Australian study, the risk of uterine rupture from oxytocin was found to be much higher than that from a previous cesarean scar.[104] Even more important, the risk of death is much lower for vaginal deliveries following surgical delivery than it is for repeat cesarean sections.

> Using the *best* results reported today, maternal mortality with repeat cesarean section is 10/10,000. In contrast, the *worst* results from a trial of labor show maternal mortality at 0.024/10,000 [italics added].[105]

Financial risks. The cost of a cesarean delivery is much higher than the cost of a normal delivery. In 1981, private hospitals in Maryland charged $330 per day for mothers only. Mothers stayed 6.6 days, on the average, bringing the total charge to $2179.[106] Florida Blue Cross/Blue Shield reports an average charge of $500 per day for 1981.[107] In 1983, the University of Florida teaching hospital charged mothers $725 for the first day and $500 for each day thereafter, bringing the total average charge for a stay of 6.6 days to $3525.[108]

Nursery charges are additional. In 1981, for Maryland hospitals, these charges ranged from $20 to $93,755, with an average of $716 for a stay of 4.4 days.[106] However, babies born by cesarean section are much more likely than normally delivered babies to be placed in the intensive care unit (ICU) nursery, where per day charges are considerably higher and stays considerably longer than for the normal nursery. The national average charge for neonatal ICUs is reported to be $15,000,[109] but is higher than that in many hospitals. At one teaching hospital, the average neonatal ICU charge is $88,000, and charges in excess of $100,000 are no longer rarities.

Another financial risk to consider is that future deliveries will be as expensive as the present one if U.S. obstetricians adhere to their policy of "once a cesarean, always a cesarean."

The expenses may continue into the recovery period, since help may be needed in the form of housekeeper/maid. In addition, the relatively long recovery period may cause loss of income for working mothers.

Reasons for the Increase in Cesarean Sections

Why are there so many surgical deliveries? Why has the cesarean section rate increased so much in recent years? There are many contributing factors. One, already discussed, is the medical policy of routine repeat surgical deliveries without a "trial of labor." Another, also noted earlier, is the daisy chain effect of hospitals' interventionist technologies. Most hospitals require electronic fetal monitoring, and electronic fetal monitoring increase the likelihood of surgical delivery (see p. 9). Hospital personnel routinely administer painkilling drugs; in addition to killing pain, these drugs slow labor, cause hypertension, and have other effects, all of which also increase the likelihood of surgical delivery. Similarly, a horizontal position, artificial induction of labor, and other technological interventions all serve to convert low-risk pregnancies into deliveries at high risk for surgery.

A third reason for the tremendous increase in the cesarean section rate stems from changes in this country's obstetrical residency training programs. According to a survey of 100 of the nation's leading (and older) obstetricians,[6] yesterday's graduates learned the art of obstetrics, for example, how to turn a breech (feet first) presentation to a cephalic (head first) presentation, whereas today's graduates learn only the technology of obstetrics, for example, the intervention procedures, including surgical delivery. In other words, current training practices may lead obstetrical graduates to convert normal, low-risk deliveries into abnormal, high-risk deliveries.

A fourth factor contributing to the escalating cesarean section rate is that the principal reasons for operating rest on subjective judgments, and obstetricians' subjective judgments have changed in recent years. Mothers of the 1980s are not laboring more slowly than mothers of the 1920s. What has changed are obstetricians' arbitrary definitions of slow labor, cephalocaudal disproportion, fetal distress, and other so-called medical indications for cesarean delivery. After analyzing cesarean section rate data for the state of New York, Dr. Andrew Fleck, Director of the Division of Maternal and Child Health, concluded,

> What we've been able to show is that Cesarean section is a provider attribute and not an attribute of the woman. . . . In other words . . . the data in

my report offers indirect evidence that the performance of a Cesarean section is unrelated to the woman's condition.[110]

Another reason for the upsurge in surgical deliveries may be economic. For more than a decade, the birth rate has been decreasing. During the same period, the number of obstetricians has been increasing. By 1978, there was already a "glut" of obstetricians/gynecologists—24,000 practicing in the United States and another 4500 residents looking forward to entering that field.[111,112] One San Antonio obstetrician was quoted as saying, "Imagine my surprise when I learned that 24 Ob/Gyns had opened offices in San Antonio in the same month. I immediately wondered: How can all these people make it?"[112] (As a matter of fact, the rate of increase of obstetricians/gynecologists in San Antonio is greater than the rate of increase of the population as a whole for that city.[112]) This can only mean that the number of billable patient procedures per obstetrician has decreased. In fact, each practicing obstetrician performed 261 deliveries in 1963, but only 145 deliveries in 1975.[6] What will happen by the end of this decade when, according to government projections, there will be an even greater surplus of obstetricians?[113]

Like other people, obstetricians have bills to pay. Faced with the prospect of declining income, how do obstetricians meet their obligations? One solution is to increase the charge to each patient. By 1980, U.S. obstetricians/gynecologists were charging $30.70 for a first office visit, $19.04 for succeeding office visits, and $27.03 for each hospital visit.[114] However, third-party reimbursement sources (private and governmental medical insurers) put a ceiling on reimbursable charges for each procedure, and this in turn put a ceiling on increasing per-visit charges.

Another solution to the income problem is to increase the number of expensive procedures such as cesarean sections. That this may have happened is suggested in the recently released federal report analyzing the reasons for the phenomenal rise in cesarean births. Doctors' fees for surgical delivery are about twice as high as for vaginal delivery.[6,115] Thus, it is theoretically possible for obstetricians to maintain the same income on only a fraction of the patient load if they do cesarean sections on most of their patients. Does this happen in practice? In 1978, the cesarean section rate for U.S. physicians with a primary practice in gynecology was 54%.[116] In the same year, a New York state survey revealed one obstetrician who delivered two thirds of his patients surgically.[5]

In reality, however, obstetricians' incomes have not remained the same. They have doubled in the last decade, from an average net income of $53,200 in 1972[114] to $105,140 in 1982.[117] Formerly among the lower paid medical specialists, obstetricians now enjoy one of the highest incomes, second only to that of surgeons and anesthesiologists. Thus it may not be a coincidence that cesarean section became one of the ten most frequently performed operative procedures by 1976.[114] A similar conclusion was drawn by the President of the American Society of Internal Medicine, who recently stated his concern that the growing surplus of physicians will ". . . increase the amount of nonessential care to ensure an adequate income in a highly competitive market."[118]

Part of the medical/economic problem is that most physicians' incomes come from the number of procedures they perform ("fee for service") rather than a straight salary. Taking note of this, the Marieskind report[6] recommends that physicians charge a standard fee for childbirth, regardless of delivery mode, which would have a restraining effect on unnecessary cesarean deliveries and would dispel charges that economic gain is a prime incentive in the decision to deliver babies surgically. However, the same recommendation was made in 1933 by the White House conference on childbirth mortality and morbidity, and the recommendation went unheeded.[1] (There is evidence from other countries as well that paying surgeons a fee for service rather than a salary markedly increases the amount of surgery they perform.[119]) The contribution of economic incentives to the rising cesarean section rate can also be inferred from the fact that the rate for women covered by Blue Cross (20.2%) is almost twice as high as the rate for women whom the doctor cannot charge (11.9%) for one reason or another.[89]

A final reason for the soaring cesarean section rate is that, from the obstetrician's point of view, everyone else is doing it, and there's safety in numbers. The patients of obstetrician-gynecologists are frequently unhappy with their physicians. In the 1-year period from July 1975 to June 1976, 20,631 of these unhappy patients sued their obstetrician-gynecologists; 8376 won their cases and collected $149 million. Currently, there are ten times more successful malpractice suits brought against obstetricians/gynecologists than against the average physician.[120] The rate of recovery against obstetricians is 42%, or the third highest of any specialty.[121] Obstetricians' major defense in anticipation of such a suit is to conform to a *standard of care*. If they do so, they cannot be found negligent. Thus, for example, from their point of view, if all other obstetricians in the area are performing 100% repeat cesarean sections, they are placing themselves in legal jeopardy by allowing a trial of labor for a woman who has had a previous cesarean birth. There is safety in numbers but risk if you go it alone.

Emotional and Psychological Risks and Benefits

The preceding section discussed physical risks and benefits of intervention procedures in terms of scientific criteria. A similar discussion of emotional and psychological risks and benefits is not possible because these topics have been neglected in scientific studies. Modern obstetrics has concerned itself with physiological variables while ignoring the psychological.[122] However, from demographic and clinical sources, there is reason to believe that emotional and psychological risks are fully as important as physical risks.

For a demographic example, one investigator points out that while postpartum depression afflicts 10% to 25% of mothers who give birth in the hospitals of industrialized countries, it is unknown in preliterate societies.[121] Clinical sources typically reveal vaguely defined but strongly held feelings of distress and repugnance, as illustrated in these brief accounts written by unhappy mothers. "The horrors of the labor-delivery room experience . . . left me with emotional scars that are still unhealed."[123] "I have had very bad experiences with hospitals and doctors with each of my children. The worst was with my last child that has caused me much fear. . . . For months I woke up with nightmares. It affected my attitude with our new baby for a long time."[124] "The technological birth, with its tension and fear for the mother and baby, the presence of drugs and, most importantly, the separation of mother and baby at birth, has made childbirth a feared torture that one must 'go through' in order to have children."[125]

The most frequent specific complaints that mothers have about the emotional and psychological effects of hospitalization and intervention procedures are that:

- They feel dehumanized.
- They are made to feel that delivery is an illness and that they are sick.
- They lose control over the situation (and for childbirth-educated mothers, this includes loss of control over breathing).
- They suffer a great loss of self-esteem.
- They become vulnerable to feelings of fear (and fear-accentuated pain), depression, and guilt.

- They feel cheated in being treated as nonentities when the obstetrician takes the limelight and adulation that should be theirs.
- They feel a loss of sexual attractiveness because of the unnatural, ugly, and invasive procedures perpetrated on their bodies (for example, from shaving or from the pain and scars of surgical procedures).[126]
- They feel that bonding has been insufficient or has been interfered with, including the establishment of new affectional ties to the baby and the restrengthening of old ties of love and affection to the husband.

The Technological Daisy Chain

As the reader will have noticed by now, obstetrical interventions are not independent of each other. On the contrary, one leads to the other, so that accepting the first intervention increases the probability that a second intervention will become "necessary," which in turn increases the probability of a third, and so on. This daisy chain of cumulative risk is illustrated in Fig. 1. One physician described this process of being pulled out to sea by the undertow of cumulative interventions after putting one foot in to test the water as follows:

> The major problem we have with these technical advances is that they encourage us to take unwarranted risks, and one intervention leads to another. We can induce labor, because it's so convenient, but then we have to monitor the contractions electronically. If the contractions are too weak, we have to increase the rate of the oxytocin infusion. When they get too strong, we have to give Demerol or an epidural to relieve the pain. If the fetus becomes distressed, as it so often does, thank goodness we have the fetal monitor to recognize the distress, and we can do an emergency Caesarean to relieve it. Then, if the baby is depressed, we have a really excellent intensive care nursery in the neonatal unit to look after him. That's a good thing, because we need it often.[127]

Separation and Bonding

Since babies born in-hospital frequently need intensive care nurseries, we should look at the effect of early separation on the bonding that is so important to the development of a strong parent-child relationship.

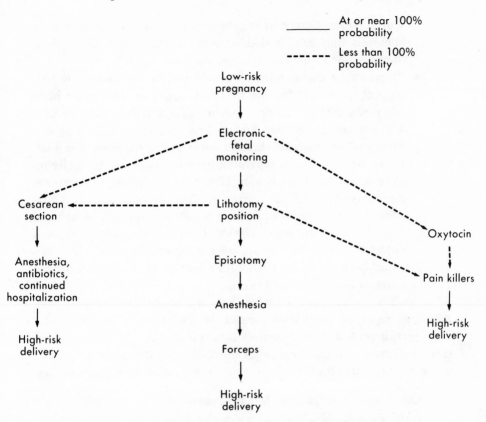

Fig. 1 Intervention Daisy Chain.

When a mother delivers at home or in a freestanding birth center, she keeps her baby with her continuously. When she delivers in a hospital, she relinquishes her baby to the hospital nursery and sees it, as a visitor, two to three times a day. This apparently trivial difference between in-hospital and out-of-hospital births may have, in reality, profound and long-lasting effects on mother, on baby, and particularly on the bonding relationship between mother and baby.

Bonding is the first step in emotional attachment of parent to infant. The essentials of bonding are extended physical contact between mother and baby, beginning immediately after birth.

- "Extended" means that after birth, mother and infant remain together and are not separated as most hospitals require.
- "Physical contact" refers to a hands-on, skin-to-skin experience. It means more than just the mother's looking at the baby. Re-

search shows that mother monkeys soon lose interest in their babies if they are denied physical contact with them, even though their visual contact is unlimited.

- "Beginning immediately after birth" means that there may be a "sensitive period" for the first few hours or days after birth when bonding is facilitated. After that, bonding may become difficult. Every farmer knows how important this sensitive period is for many nonhuman species. For example, the goat, sheep, or cow who is separated from her newborn typically rejects that young one if they later have the chance to reunite. Though evidence from human studies is less clear cut, it suggests that the same process is at work for people. At least most mothers feel that way, as evidenced in this excerpt from a mother's letter: "It was six days after birth before I saw my child, because of the difficulties he had. And it's taken three years to build our relationship."

Bonding is not restricted to mothers and babies. Fathers bond, too. Although there has been less research on the paternal side of parent-child attachment, available studies indicate that the principles of extended physical contact beginning immediately after birth are as important for father-infant bonding as they are for mother-infant bonding.

Consequences of Mother-Infant Separation

What happens to mother and baby when they are separated after birth? A considerable amount of research points to several short-term consequences. Among separated mothers, fewer breastfeed and more experience difficulties in caring for their babies.[128] Separated babies cry more and show widely fluctuating, stress-like patterns in respiration, heart rate, and temperature maintenance.[128] They gain less weight and have a higher rate of infection.[129]

Documented long-term consequences of early mother-infant separation include fewer affectionate, protective, and nurturing behaviors in mothers, as well as less self-confidence in their ability to care for their infants. These mothers also breastfeed for a shorter period and have weaker relationships with their husbands.[129] Early separated infants may even score lower on tests of intelligence and language.[129]

In addition to bonding problems, mother-infant separation means that newborns will be placed in newborn nurseries and thus exposed to all the risks there, principally infection. Over and above the risk of disease, giving up one's newborn child means giving up control over the events and happenings in that child's life. In a teaching-affiliated hospital, there is the likelihood that some researcher will use the baby as a subject without obtaining informed parental consent.[130] In any hospital, there is the possibility, albeit rare, of mistaken identification.[131]

A Special Note on Risks to Babies

Hospital birth carries many risks for babies as well as for mothers. So many, in fact, that it would require another whole book to examine them thoroughly. Some of these risks have been mentioned in earlier sections. In this section, we list the major ones (Table 1-1) and refer concerned readers to other sources for additional information. Principal among these sources is the book, *Iatrogenic Problems in Neonatal Intensive Care.*[132]

In examining Table 1-1, notice that many of the risks for the baby stem from interventions that have been imposed on the mother. For example, all drugs and medications given to the mother before, during, and after delivery (if she breastfeeds) increase the risk for the baby. Also, any maternal intervention that increases the likelihood of preterm delivery also increases the likelihood of the baby being placed in the intensive care unit (sometimes called "maximum care unit"), where risks are greater than in normal newborn nurseries. Cesarean sections provide an example of such an intervention.

In addition to the indirectly imposed risks for the baby, hospitalization itself involves a whole set of directly imposed risks for the baby. One is the risk from infectious bacteria that periodically sweep through nurseries. Infection rates are particularly high for intensive care units and for teaching hospitals, as compared to regular hospital nurseries: "University hospitals with neonatal intensive care units have rates as high as 24 per cent."[133] Why? Among other reasons is that hospital personnel, according to a recent study,[134] simply fail to wash their hands after touching one patient and before touching the next. The study found that "physicians were among the worst offenders."[134,135]

Infection rates are also higher (by about 300%) in university, county, and city hospitals than in community and federal hospitals.[135] Both illness and death rates are substantially higher for hospital-born babies than for planned home births, an unfortunate statistic that is discussed in the next chapter.

Table 1.1   Risks Associated with Hospital Nurseries

Procedure or Intervention	Risk
Risks for babies admitted to any hospital nursery	
Admission to an experimental study as a subject for research	Failure to get informed consent from parents
	Other risks depend on nature of research
Admission to nursery	Diseases associated with hospital nurseries, e.g., staph infection; *Klebsiella* (infectious intestinal bacteria); adenovirus type 7; Q fever; Legionnaire's disease; meningitis
	Deprivation of cuddling and maternal contact
Circumcision	Pain
	Irritability
	Damage to penis
	Infection
	Psychological trauma
	Death
Exposure to high noise levels from incubators and other nursery equipment, other babies, and nursery staff	Damage to ears, hearing
Formula, sugar water	Lowering of natural immunity to disease, illness
	Allergies
Handling (up to 185 times in 24 hours)	Disturbed rest and sleep; fatigue
	Increased risk of exposure to infection
Indirect exposure to drugs through mother's milk	Teratogenic, toxic exposure
Separation from mother	Interference with bonding
Silver nitrate in eyes	Swelling and closure of eyelids
	Interference with bonding
Vitamin K injection	Separation of red blood cells
	Jaundice
Risks for babies admitted to maximum or intensive care nursery	
Blood transfusion	Immediate complications: air embolism, sepsis, cardiac failure, cardiac arrhythmias, hypothermia, hyperkalemia, hypocalcemia, hypomagnesemia, citrate toxicity, metabolic acidosis, and hypoglycemia
	Delayed complications: hepatitis, cytomegalic virus disease, *Plasmodium*

Table 1.1 Risks Associated with Hospital Nurseries—cont'd

Procedure or Intervention	Risk
	vivax infections, hepatic cirrhosis, portal hypertension
Catheterization (plastic tube in artery)	Thrombosis (blood clot)
	Death (3-4/1000)
	Infection (80% after 24 hours)
	Umbilical artery spasm and perforation
	Loss of fingertips, hand, or lower arm
	Interference with bonding
Drugs, directly administered (babies in ICUs receive an average of 7, as high as 21). Some of the more common drugs and their effects are:	
Antacid (e.g., sodium bicarbonate; THAM)	Blood in urine
	Intracranial hemorrhage
	Bladder degeneration
	Excessive sodium in blood
Antibiotic	Gray syndrome (baby turns gray)
Anticoagulant (thins blood)	Hemorrhage (loss of blood)
Anticonvulsant (for fits and seizures)	Central nervous system depression
Calcium	Cardiac arrest (heart stops beating)
Cardiac glycoside (e.g., digitalis)	Arrhythmia (irregular heartbeat)
Electrolyte (potassium, magnesium, phosphate, sulfate, bicarbonate, sodium)	Excessive amount in blood
Glucose	Tissue degeneration
Intravenous fluids	In excess, congestive heart failure
	Scar tissue
Sedative	Central nervous system depression
	Respiratory arrest (stops breathing)
	Loss of sucking response; feeding problems
Vasopressor	Tachycardia (fast heartbeat)
Electronic monitoring devices, external (respiration, heart, etc.)	Wrong diagnosis and therapy following operator error in using and reading equipment
	Equipment failure
	Shock
Intravenous and tube feeding	Acidosis
	Depletion of blood phosphorous followed by anemia and impaired oxygen transport

Continued.

Table 1.1   Risks Associated with Hospital Nurseries—cont'd

Procedure or Intervention	Risk
Intravenous and tube feeding—cont'd	
	Elevated blood ammonia levels
	Impaired peripheral nerve function
	Acute neurological disturbance
	Abnormally rapid and disproportionate head growth
	Liver dysfunction
	Depletion of copper, zinc, and essential fatty acids
	Staph infection and diarrhea
	Death from aspiration of food
	Interference with bonding
Neglect (from high nurse-to-baby ratio)	Delayed treatment of problems
	Psychological trauma
	Sensory deprivation
Oxygen	In large quantities, retrolental fibroplasia (formation of fibrous tissue behind crystalline lens of eye)—partial or total blindness
	Bronchopulmonary dysplasia ("respirator lung")
Phototherapy (light ray treatment)	Diarrhea
	Decreased weight gain
	Decreased blood platelet count
	Interference with bonding (baby's eye patches)
	Inflammation of conjunctivae (lining of eyelids and eyeballs) from eye patches
Radiant heaters	Shock
	Effects of infrared radiation unknown
Radiation, x-ray	Interference with normal central nervous system development
	Increased risk of later cancer and sterility

2

Why Interventions?

From the information presented in the previous chapter, several conclusions can be drawn about interventions:

- They are an entrenched aspect of hospital birth and apparently unavoidable, so that choosing to deliver in-hospital means choosing high-tech birth.
- Most interventions were initially adopted for use in high-risk births but have gradually taken over low-risk births as well.
- For women with normal pregnancies, interventions pose more risks than benefits.
- Some interventions, for example, fetal monitors, have been evaluated by research that for the most part is methodologically unsound. Nevertheless, hospitals still use these interventions.
- Some interventions, for example, shaving, have been evaluated in scientifically sound research and found to be more risky than beneficial. They are used anyway.
- Some interventions, for example, episiotomy, have been evaluated inadequately, if at all, but are still a routine part of hospital practice.
- In sum, interventions rest on faith rather than on research evidence concerning their safety and effectiveness. Others rest on research evidence that is inappropriate or unsound.

In view of all this negative evidence, the logical questions are why so many interventions continue to be used in low-risk births and why some are used at all. Since there is no sound scientific basis for imposing technology on healthy women undergoing normal labor and delivery, why do medical personnel do so? Since the risks of interventions outweigh their benefits for normal birth, why do physicians insist on using them? There are several reasons. None of them is medical; none of them is appealing.

A major reason for using technological interventions is that they serve financial and economic interests. Interventions are big business. Consider drugs, for example. Drugs are the most widely used form of therapy in the United States. In 1981, drugs cost us $21 billion, almost 1% of the gross national product.[1] In 1980, pharmacists filled 1.4 billion prescriptions[2] — more than five prescriptions for every person living in the United States. In addition to prescription drugs, the FDA estimates that there are a half million different over-the-counter products being marketed, with annual sales of $6 billion in 1981.[3]

Like any other business, the health industry's first priority is to make money. If it does not show a profit, it will not stay in business. Hospitals are not charities. Physicians are not philanthropists. Manufacturers of health products are not benevolent societies. They all must pay salaries to themselves and their staffs, mortgages and rents, stockholders' dividends, taxes, insurance, and so on. (Malpractice insurance rates for obstetricians are now over $40,000 a year in some states.)

Technology is profitable all the way around — for manufacturers, for hospitals, and for medical staff. Manufacturers of fetal monitors, for example, collected $25 million in 1976 and $30 million in 1978. They anticipate sales of $40 million by 1986.[4] As one obstetrician remarked, in surveying the technological scene, "the quality of an obstetrical service has become judged . . . by the number of fetal monitors it has available. We have all . . . become slaves to the technological environment."[5]

Hospitals gain financially from using technology because all interventions yield billable charges. A prime example is the cesarean section. The hospital profits in one respect because the hospital stay after cesarean birth is twice as long as after normal delivery. In addition, surgical delivery allows the hospital to add many extra charges to its bill, including operating room, recovery room, surgical supplies, anesthetic supplies, pharmacy supplies, intravenous equipment, blood and transfusion equipment, laboratory work, oxygen, and x-ray examinations.[6] Along with the x-ray and laboratory departments, its in-patient pharmacy is the hospital's big money-maker. Hospitals buy pharmaceuticals at wholesale cost but resell them to patients at marked-up "dosage charges." We asked one university-affiliated teaching hospital pharmacy in an average cost-of-living region what it pays and what it charges for some of the medications most commonly used in obstetrics.

Table 2.1 Typical Hospital Pharmacy Costs and Charges

Pharmacy Item	Wholesale Price Paid by Hospital	Dosage Charge to Obstetrical In-Patient
Set-up (stand and tubing) for 1 liter intravenous fluid (5% dextrose + water)	$.78	$19.95
Oxytocin (administered through IV fluid; for total cost, add $5.85 + $19.95)	.26	5.85
Meperidine (Demerol) for pain—50 mg injection	.30	6.95
2 Tylenol tablets	.01	1.00
1 oz Milk of Magnesia (each ounce separately packaged)	.17	2.45

Table 2-1 itemizes these costs. Many items are billed whether or not they are used; for example, even if the patient does not need a transfusion, she is billed for having transfusion equipment set up and ready to be used.

Medical staff profit from use of technological interventions because they are directly involved in applying the intervention or because they are indirectly involved in coping with the complications resulting from use of the intervention. In either event, their services are billable to the patient. Surgical delivery again provides an example. Instead of a single medical person "catching" the vaginally delivered baby, cesarean section means that additional physicians participate in the delivery, including an anesthesiologist, an assistant surgeon, and maybe a perinatologist. Each of them bills the patient. In addition, the chief obstetrician bills the patient at a higher rate than for vaginal delivery.[7] The rate is substantial: obstetrics is now the third highest paid medical specialty.[8]

Closely allied to technology's financial profit is its temporal profit. Technology saves time. For the physician, time and money are interchangeable. For example, the obstetrician used to have to listen through a stethoscope for the baby's heart rate. Today, the electronic fetal monitor automatically detects and records the baby's heart rate, freeing the physician or nurse to do other things. As another example, normal labor, during which a nurse or physician must attend the mother, may take 15 to 20 hours. Surgical delivery, however, takes only 15 to 20 minutes, thus saving the physician a very substantial amount of time.

Oxytocin is another time-saver. As one mother complained in a letter to her obstetrician: "As it was you still turned the drip up too high. My labor lasted 3 hours. As your medical books will tell you that is not a normal length of time particularly for a woman whose two previous labors lasted 36 and 18 hours."

Another reason hospitals use technology is quite simply that it is present and available. Availability of equipment, of space, and of staff becomes a psychological commitment to their use—quite apart from economic considerations—so that, like dependent children, their presence in the hospital "family" requires the generation of additional income to support them. An unused fetal monitor is a tacit admission that the chief of obstetrics exercised poor judgment in spending $10,000. An empty hospital room on the obstetrics ward is an invitation to "squatters" from other, overcrowded departments. The hospital's decision to add a staff member in a new and very narrow specialty, for example, a *perinatologist*, means that something must be found for that physician to do. It is demoralizing, indeed unthinkable, for a physician to have nothing to do—to be, as it were, unwanted. For these very reasons, experts predict that technology will increase as the birth rate decreases.[9] They also predict that technology will increase as the number of obstetricians increases. (The government forecast is for a 10,000 surplus by 1990.[10]) The education of obstetricians formalizes their commitments to rely on intervention as their obstetrical model. As one observer commented, "During training, the physician learns that technology is there to be used, or rather, that the technology is to be used because it is there.[11]

Other psychological reasons have been advanced for hospitals' reliance on technology. One is that they make obstetricians feel more important and enhance their image. As one reflective physician remarked, "The doctor replaces the parents as the star in the drama of birth, and patterns of interference in birthing are inevitable."[12] We Americans value technology as good; by extension, we also see as good those people who know how to use that technology. The more hardware obstetricians impose on delivery, the more skills they bring to bear—even if all are unnecessary—the more their goodliness approaches godliness.

Gods traditionally keep their distance from non-gods, and so it is with physicians. Obstetricians strive to remain uninvolved, and technological hardware helps them do that.

> Modern equipment . . . makes it so easy for the professional—the doctor or nurse—to remain uninvolved. It's so easy to pay attention to the ma-

chine, instead of the woman or the couple. The baby becomes a product, to be produced in the most efficient way, and as long as her apgar score is good, we can feel we have been successful.[12]

The machine is useful because it discourages both intimacy and communication; it allows the physician to remain aloof. Drugs are also useful because they ensure that the patient doesn't demand involvement. Nurses and doctors are liberal dispensers of sedatives, tranquilizers, and anesthetics in part because it distresses them if their patients become distressed.[12]

In addition, interventions help justify the physician's large professional fees and small expenditures of time with patients. For the most part, obstetricians spend no time at all with their patients during labor and very little time with them during delivery. Sometimes they do not make it to the delivery room at all. The standing order prescriptions, the mechanical gadgets, the ritualistic preparations such as enemas and shaving—all appear as extensions of obstetricians and emanations of their presence even in their absence. In other words, interventions make patients less likely to question the propriety of paying $1500 for 15 minutes' service.

Still another reason why medical staff rely heavily on technology is their conviction that practicing medicine the way other physicians practice it ("standard of care") is the best legal protection against malpractice suits. For example, two recent surveys[6] sought prominent obstetricians' opinions about the reasons for soaring cesarean section rates in the United States. The reason most frequently given was threat of a malpractice suit. Doing what other physicians do is a persuasive legal argument. It means, however, that the decision to use an intervention is determined by legal criteria rather than by medical criteria. As one critic remarked, "Medicine is a discipline of opinion where 'accepted practice' is determined by a majority professional vote, not by the scientific method."[13]

Another reason for physicians' reliance on technological interventions stems from their training. In a recent government study on the rise in cesarean section rates, prominent obstetricians frequently cited training as a chief reason for the increase. Obstetrical residents are no longer being taught normal obstetrics. As one physician commented, "The average resident today, trained in our most modern institutions, graduates ill-prepared to manage clinically many obstetric conditions and feels literally that he cannot practice without the presence of a fetal monitor at his fingertips."[5] Residents learn how to use mechanical gadgets rather than manual skills, how to extract babies surgically rather than vaginally, and how to use drugs rather than nondrug alternatives for pain. All obstetricians interviewed in that government study stressed the importance of the department chairperson in shaping training policy and practice for medical students and residents.[6] In defense of their policies, department chairpersons protest that applicants for residency training demand substantial practice with interventions, including fetal monitoring, amniocentesis, and, most importantly, surgery. They complain that only by emphasizing intervention training can they attract good residents.

Most technological interventions were created for use with those few high-risk mothers and babies who might otherwise die. Nevertheless, as we have seen, there are many reasons for using technological interventions that have nothing to do with high risk and saving lives: financial profit for manufacturers, hospitals, and medical staff; saving professionals' time; commitment to use technological interventions just because they are available; physician's ego gratification; protection against involvement; justification of high professional fees; anticipated defense against malpractice suits; and lack of professional training in normal obstetrics.

So many and so compelling are these reasons that they, rather than the patient's true risk status, have come to determine the use of technological interventions. In fact, to rationalize the use of technological interventions, obstetricians now declare that all mothers and babies are high risk. Physicians are quoted as saying, "No pregnancy or birth is normal except in retrospect."[14] "Because labor is a stress to the fetus, the intrapartum period is a hazardous time of life, and perhaps all infants should be considered at high risk during this time."[15]

• • •

Why has hospital obstetrics relied on interventions when they are inappropriate—indeed, dangerous—for low-risk births? Why have some interventions been adopted on the basis of faith and belief rather than on scientific evidence of their safety and effectiveness? We have explored and identified some reasons for hospitals' and obstetricians' insistence on using high technology interventions, including:
- Interventions are financially profitable.
- Interventions save time.
- Interventions are often used because they are present and available.

- Interventions provide a vehicle for some physicians' ego trips.
- Interventions are a means by which physicians can remain uninvolved.
- Interventions "justify" some obstetricians' charging large fees for small expenditures of patient contact time.
- Obstetricians believe that interventions protect them against malpractice suits.
- High-tech birth is the only kind most obstetricians know.

Technology has warped some physicians' view of pregnancy and birth. As one mother commented, "Before the hospital thing pregnancy was a *normal, nice* condition. I'm not so sure it isn't an *illness* now."[14]

3

Birth Centers:
An Alternative to Hospital
and Home Birth

The childbirth movement of the 1970s and parent demand for another way of birth precipitated the emergence of an entirely new idea—the freestanding birth center. Here at last was a birthplace for families who wanted neither high-technology birth in the hospital nor low-technology birth in the home. They wanted something in between. The significance of this innovation to maternity care, how birth centers have developed, and what they offer to childbearing families will be described in this chapter.

The birth center has been defined as a short-stay, homelike facility that is not physically attached to a hospital, in other words, a "freestanding" birthplace. It provides full maternity and gynecological services for healthy women who are expecting to have a normal pregnancy and birth. Qualified health professionals, that is, nurse-midwives and physicians who have access to a nearby hospital should the need arise, provide prenatal, birth, postpartum, and newborn care to women and their families.

Birth centers are not "mini-hospitals," nor are they an adaptation of the hospital.[1] On the contrary, they are an adaptation of the home. Only healthy, low-risk women are eligible to have their babies in birth centers, since they are not equipped for high-technology childbirth, as is the acute care hospital. Therefore, every birth center uses rigid

46

screening and selection procedures for families before enrolling them in the birth center program.

In most birth centers, a health team consisting of nurse-midwives, obstetricians, pediatrician, public health nurse, and other support staff provide care for families. If a change or complication occurs in a woman's health during pregnancy, labor, or delivery that makes her ineligible to continue at the birth center, she is referred for physician care and hospital delivery.[1]

The birth center is a place for the entire family, where children, grandparents, family members, and friends are welcomed and encouraged to learn about and take part in the birth. Pregnancy and birth are treated as normal and healthy processes in the birth center, in contrast to the sickness and medical orientation in the hospital. The family shares in decisions and choices about their childbirth experience. Special attention is given to the emotional and social aspects of childbirth as events to be shared and celebrated by those people who are most important to the mother.

Why Birth Centers?

In the early 1970s, many women began to express their feelings of dissatisfaction and rejection for the hospital way of birth. It was the beginning of the out-of-hospital birth movement. Home births were increasing, and at the same time some maternity organizations and professionals were looking for ways to bridge the gap between hospital and home birth. The public wanted a maternity service that was safe, economical, personalized, and family oriented. And so, in 1975 the first birth center opened in New York City under the direction of the Maternity Center Association. It was named The Childbearing Center, and this birth center has served as the model for others around the country.

Since then, the birth center concept has been growing in leaps and bounds, changing permanently the way that maternity care is provided. But opening the doors of birth centers has been far from easy. Opposition has been strong from some obstetricians, organized medical groups, hospitals, and others. Underlying this resistance is the medical community's fear of economic competition in an expanding maternity marketplace overflowing with physicians.

From a mere handful of birth centers in the United States in the mid-1970s, the number has grown to over 100 by mid-1983, with 350 more in the planning stages.[2] Suddenly, state and regional public health and planning agencies were faced with the job of licensing and setting standards of care for an entirely new type of health facility, for which no guidelines and standards had been designed.

It quickly became obvious that a central resource and support system for birth centers was needed, and in 1981 the Maternity Center Association once again took the lead and created the Cooperative Birth Center Network. This body has now been renamed the National Association of Childbearing Centers. The job of this organization was to "assist and support the development and accessibility of safe, cost-efficient birth alternatives, with particular attention to the out-of-hospital birth center."[3]

To clear the way for the future growth of birth centers, the Maternity Center Association was awarded a grant in which it undertook to do the following:

- Promote a wider public understanding of the birth center concept.
- Create a cooperative resource and information network for dissemination of the model at the operational level.
- Develop standards or recommendations for regulation for the guidance of public health officials, policy planners, and insurance carriers.[1]

The momentum for establishing birth centers has increased rapidly under the encouragement of the National Association of Childbearing Centers. Requests for information, consultation, assistance, and support have poured in from interested midwives, physicians, parents, and consumer childbirth groups. Regional workshops have been conducted around the country to provide information on the financing, managing, operating, and marketing of birth centers.

At the same time, the Association was concerned that regulations be established to ensure quality care and conduct of birth centers. The Association believed it was essential that these facilities be licensed, as are all health facilities, so that certain minimum standards for safety would be met. The birth center's license would need to include construction of the facility, qualifications of the personnel working in it, and requirements for its safe operation. Early in 1982 this step was advanced with the publication of "Information for Establishing Standards or Regulations for Free Standing Birth Centers."[4] These guidelines serve as a model for health regulatory agencies, such as state health departments, whose job it is to write standards, guidelines, and regulations for birth centers.

The American Public Health Association (APHA) was the first national health agency to make a formal policy statement endorsing birth centers in November, 1982, when it published "Guidelines for Licensing and Regulating Birth Centers."[5] It took the following supportive position:

- Some women are seeking alternatives to the acute care hospital for normal pregnancy and birth.
- Birth centers in and out of hospitals can offer this alternative to women and their families.
- Births to healthy mothers can occur safely in birth centers outside the setting of an acute care hospital.
- These births can be safely and competently attended by professionals trained specifically in the conduct of normal, uncomplicated childbirth, and early recognition of complications or abnormalities of labor.
- Birth centers have a potential for reducing the costs of maternity care.
- The American Public Health Association adopted a position, in October 1979, that endorsed family-centered maternity care, demonstration projects for alternatives in maternity care, and research in this area.
- State and local jurisdictions have been called upon to regulate birth centers.
- The APHA has a public responsibility and an organizational commitment to ensure that standards exist to protect the health, safety, and welfare of mothers and infants.[5]

In contrast to the APHA position, The American College of Obstetricians and Gynecologists (ACOG) issued a policy statement in December, 1982, in which it once again took its traditional stand against out-of-hospital birth.[6] Its statement on alternative birth centers is as follows:

The hospital setting provides the safest atmosphere for mother, fetus, and infant during labor, delivery, and in the postpartum period. Birth centers, within the hospital complex and functioning under the protocols of the Department of Obstetrics and Gynecology, provide safeguards to ensure similar safety. Scientific methodology to investigate outcome of normal delivery adequately has been problematic as documented in a National Academy of Sciences study[7] and until scientific studies are available to evaluate safety and outcome in free-standing alternative birth centers, such centers cannot be encouraged. There may be exceptional geographically isolated situations where special programs are necessary.[6]

Organized pediatrics, namely the American Academy of Pediatrics, has also aligned itself with this position.[8]

It seems certain, however, that birth centers are here to stay and are becoming an integral part of the expanding movement toward ambulatory health care facilities. Already by mid-1983, more than a dozen states have passed legislation licensing birth centers and many more are working on the necessary legislation.[2] Insurance carriers, such as Blue Cross/Blue Shield and Medicaid, now reimburse families for birth center services in most places.

Since 1975, five birth centers have had to close their doors.[9] Reasons include (1) insufficient start-up funds and assessment of the market, (2) inability to obtain reimbursement for the services provided, (3) no licensure (which affected the birth center's ability to obtain reimbursement), and (4) difficulty in obtaining staff.[9] This closure rate, amounting to 4.5% of the total birth centers, indicates surprising strength in the small-business world. Birth centers have held their own and multiplied in the "highly competitive and often antagonistic marketplace."[9]

Birth Center Philosophy in Action

Earlier we described the hospital way of conducting birth. The normal, healthy process of birth most women experience is frequently transformed into a high-risk event in the hospital. The woman in labor is treated like a sick patient from the moment she sets foot inside the hospital doors and is put into a wheelchair. The focus is not on birth as a happy, family event but as a medical procedure that relies heavily on drugs and technology. Institutional power and control take over the birth and the participants, who must conform to the hospital regulations and practices.

Progress has occurred, however. The recent establishment of birthing rooms and family-centered birth settings in the hospital now provides welcome alternatives. Other family-centered options such as rooming-in, children visiting, childbirth education, and early discharge have been introduced. Nevertheless, critics have pointed out that many families may well be shortchanged in their hospital alternative birth experience, since the promise of a family-centered philosophy and environment often is not fulfilled.[10] In their rush to offer birth alternatives, many hospitals provide what amounts to family-centered tokenism and the restrictive policies and practices still apply to all.

The freestanding birth center, on the other hand, is designed particularly around the needs of the family rather than around the needs of

Table 3.1 Comparisons of Maternity Care in a Hospital and Freestanding Birth Center

Hospital	Birth center
Provider-dominated governing board	Consumer-dominated governing board
Acute care institution	Homelike facility
Serves high- and low-risk families	Serves low-risk families
High-volume patient load	Low-volume client load
Room-to-room transfer of mother and baby	No room-to-room transfer of mother and family
Illness model of care	Prevention and health promotion model of care
Primarily physician-nurse staffing	Primarily nurse-midwife staffing with physician backup
Pathology-centered philosophy	Family-centered philosophy
Medical-technological management	Psychological-social-physiological management
Dependency role for mother	Self-help role for mother
Professional control and decision making	Joint professional-family control and decision making
High cost	Low cost

the facility. Family-centered care is a special attitude and philosophy toward birth, where the whole family is involved and shares in the event. This approach to maternity care is what makes childbirth in a birth center much more like a home birth. The family is welcomed as guests and made to feel comfortably at home and full participants in every aspect of their care. The presence of a living room, children's play area, kitchen and dining area, and library contributes to the homelike atmosphere. Table 3-1 shows the differences between a hospital and a birth center as two facilities that provide maternity care.

Since every woman and her family are different, there are no "routines" during labor and birth in the birth center. Women actively plan and participate in their care throughout pregnancy, birth, and the postpartum period. Each family, together with their nurse-midwife, develops a personalized birth plan just for them. Drugs or procedures are not used unless there is a need or indication for them. Similarly, and in keeping with the nonmedical approach, electronic fetal monitors, forceps, and chemical forms of induction or stimulation (for example, Pitocin) are not used. During labor and birth, mothers wear their own gown, get into whatever positions they find comfortable, eat and drink lightly if they wish, and have family members, including children, with them all the time.

Contrary to the hospital setting, where mothers are transferred from labor room, to delivery room, to recovery room, and finally to postpartum room, mothers stay in one place in the birth center—the bedroom where the baby is born. Birth centers honor the preference of women to labor and deliver in the same place. Research supports this preference.[11]

After birth, the baby is examined by a pediatrician in the parents' presence, and the parents begin feeding and taking care of their newborn right away with the help of their nurse-midwife. Families usually leave the birth center 12 to 24 hours after birth, and on the first day home, as well as a few days later, a public health nurse visits the family to see that all is going well. When the baby is about a week old, the family returns to the birth center for a checkup. Families are also encouraged to call as often as they need during these early weeks at home. A final visit to the birth center 6 weeks after the birth completes the program.

Safety

The primary way of ensuring safety in a birth center is its use of a careful screening process to ensure that families are low risk and therefore eligible for enrollment. The criteria for assessing the risk status of women are developed with the advice of maternity care experts, and they are applied by the professional staff to each woman during pregnancy, labor, and delivery and after birth. If any of the listed problems develops in a mother, she is referred to a birth center physician and, if necessary, transferred to a backup hospital.[1]

Another important element of safety in the birth center is provided by a maternity care system that is based on prevention and health promotion. Special attention is paid to prenatal care, nutrition, avoidance of medications, assumption of personal responsibility and self-help activities, encouragement of breastfeeding, and an extensive parent education program.

Birth centers are staffed by a professional health team whose members have carefully assigned responsibilities, thus providing another safety assurance. Nurse-midwives give most of the physical care to the childbearing women. Obstetrical specialists provide backup for the nurse-midwives. They see each family twice or more during the prenatal period and are available at other times for consultation. Nurse-midwives are trained to observe any change from the normal, and if this should occur, the backup specialist determines if physician or hospital care is necessary. Pediatricians, public health nurses, and other support staff also belong to the birth center team.

The prearranged system for emergency care provides another safety factor for the birth center. Under a formal contract with an ambulance company and nearby acute care hospital, a family (accompanied by a birth center staff member) can be quickly transferred for the necessary care. Every birth center also keeps emergency equipment on hand and ready for each birth, including oxygen, suction, infant warmer, emergency transfer bassinette, and resuscitation equipment. Practice drills are held to prepare staff in case of an emergency.

The birth center building itself must meet state and local fire, safety, and zoning standards. Facilities for sterilization, laundry, bathroom, toilet, kitchen, utility, storage, and emergency equipment are provided, in addition to the birthing rooms, family and children's rooms, reception area, library, and examination rooms.[1]

The issue of which birth setting offers the greatest safety for mother and baby continues to be a source of argument among health professionals and parents. Although a government study could not come to any firm conclusion on the matter, stating that "reliable information about the safety of different birth settings is lacking,"[7] there is in fact enough research to indicate that, as far as neonatal mortality is concerned, birth center delivery appears to be safe for low-risk families.

Studies and Surveys

Although birth centers are a recent innovation, one study has been made to examine the outcomes of 1938 women who gave birth in eleven birth centers in the United States between 1972 and 1979.[13] It was the first national collaborative study of birth centers. The average age of the women in the study was 25 years, 88% were married, 63% were white, 34% were Hispanic, and 2% were black. Certified nurse-midwives attended 79% of the women throughout labor and birth, physicians assisted 14% of the women, and graduate or student nurse-midwives assisted 5% of the women.

No drugs were used in nearly 60% of labors, 89% were spontaneous deliveries, and 5% were cesarean deliveries at the backup hospital. Of the babies, 95% were full term with an average weight of 7.7 pounds at birth, and at discharge 79% were being breastfed. After labor began, 15% of the birth center families had to be transferred to the backup hospital because of complications. The newborn death rate (*neonatal mortality*) for birth center babies (including transfers to the hospital) was 4.6 deaths per 1000 live births.[13] This rate compares very favorably with a newborn death rate of 11.6 deaths per 1000 live births nationwide in 1975 and 8.4 deaths per 1000 live births in 1980.[7]

Another study provided some operational statistics about birth centers. Toward the end of 1982, a questionnaire was sent to the 91 birth centers that were known to be in operation.[14] Of the 62 centers that replied, 50% were established as nonprofit corporations and 34.4% as private (that is, professional) corporations. The primary care provider was the nurse-midwife in 45% of the centers reporting; in 29%, both physicians and nurse-midwives provided care; and in 22%, physicians with nursing staff were in charge.

For the years 1980 to 1982, 11,622 births were reported and the average percentage of women transferred from the birth center to the hospital in labor was 13%.[14] Nonroutine medical procedures performed at the birth center included circumcision (48%), Pitocin induction (7%), forceps delivery (20.6%), vacuum extraction (7%), and cesarean section (3.4%).[14] In looking at these figures, we must remember that birth centers are designed for uncomplicated births. Therefore any trend that indicates an increase in the number of medical procedures and interventions used in birth centers should be viewed with alarm. The survey makes a strong statement concerning this potential problem: "It is important, if procedures such as Pitocin induction, Pitocin augmentation, forceps, or emergency cesarean section are proposed for use in birth centers, that these interventions be carefully evaluated before they are accepted."[14]

Individual freestanding birth centers have also been described from the perspective of their experiences in their struggle to become established, their programs, outcomes of births, and other details. These reports confirm the safety and effectiveness of this type of maternity service.[12,15,16]

Cost Savings

Birth centers have already demonstrated cost savings in maternity care. For example, in analyzing data from The Childbearing Center in New York City, Lubic notes that birth center care "is markedly less expensive than traditional hospital care for both families and the health care delivery system, while at the same time it provides safe, high-quality, personalized maternity care."[1] In fact, the average cost of a normal birth in the hospital is about double that of most birth centers.[17] In the 1982 birth center survey, the average charge for birth center services was $800, with a range from $200 to $1700.[14] The average charge for "comparable hospital care," on the other hand, was $1713, with a range from $550 to $3750.[14] Reported birth center charges average 47.7% of hospital charges for the same care.[14]

Birth centers can charge less because of the type of facility— usually a home that has been converted as needed to meet standards— and also because expensive technology and equipment are unnecessary in this setting. Another reason for low cost to the birth center family is that nurse-midwives often provide the care, and their income is about one fifth that of obstetrician-gynecologists.

Summary

To summarize, the primary contributions to maternal, newborn, and family childbirth services made by freestanding birth centers include the increase in family participation, the emphasis on prevention and health promotion, minimal medical intervention and technology, personalized and flexible care, and lower costs. This birth setting is described as being "both medically safe and psychologically secure" in a recent government report,[7] with the professional health team of nurse-midwives and physicians who staff the birth center providing a "recognized standard of care."[7]

In an increasingly high-risk and technologically oriented field, freestanding birth centers allow families to expand their choices for low-risk maternity care. As the birth center movement grows, more and more families will have access to this alternative delivery system. Furthermore, the general public will soon be able to "let their fingers do the walking" and look up "Birth Centers" as a heading in the telephone directory Yellow Pages in the United States.[18] The time of the birth center has definitely arrived!

4

Low-Tech Birth:
Home Delivery

An increasing number of mothers choose to deliver at home. Why? This chapter explores the reasons for choosing home delivery, describes benefits and risks of home delivery, and compares home and hospital in terms of exposure to interventions and overall safety for mother and child.

Home and Hospital Compared
Preference for Home Birth

Home births increased 300% between 1973 and 1980.[1] In some areas of California and Oregon, more than 10% of all planned births take place out of the hospital. The biggest contributors to this increase are not the poor and uneducated families but come straight from America's middle class. These families give as their primary reasons for choosing home birth rather than hospital birth a desire to preserve family togetherness; a conviction that hospitals, geared as they are to sick people, are psychologically and physiologically dangerous for healthy mothers and babies; an inclination to labor and deliver naturally and to avoid the high-tech interventions imposed by doctors and hospitals; a desire to stay in control of birthing and not relinquish decision making to medical personnel; a wish to avoid contact with many strangers who may treat one as inferior, incapable, and inconsequential; previous bad hospital experiences; and last, as well as least, an unwillingness to pay exorbitant sums to doctors and hospitals. Here, in their words, are the reasons home birth mothers have given for their decision:

- I'm healthy and my baby's healthy. We don't belong in a place where everyone else is diseased and ill.
- I wanted to be close to my baby and family members.
- I know my body and wanted to be in control of it. That's easier to do at home.
- Hospital interventions and routine procedures aren't always in my best interest; they often cause more harm than good.
- I feel that birth should be given back to women—myself and midwives.
- Moving to a hospital is very disrupting and interferes with the ongoing flow of labor.
- I'm intelligent and don't like being treated like an idiot.
- I distrust doctors and their "godlike" attitudes.
- I've been around animals all my life—they go where they feel comfortable and safe.
- Since drugs are more available in the hospital, I would be more likely to use them and regret it later.
- At home, I was able to use my own birth position.
- I don't like being a prisoner in the hospital—wheelchairs, straps on the delivery table, waiting to be released when you're ready to leave.
- I preferred a woman birth attendant.
- I wanted someone to help with what I was doing—not do it all themselves.
- I wanted to get to know the person delivering me.
- I am relaxed at home and have better mental control—tension causes pain and complications.
- I wanted to keep my baby with me all the time and nurse it whenever I wanted; it made me a better person and mother.
- I am bothered by the smells and germs in hospitals.
- There is too much obstetrical intervention in hospitals, like schedules, fetal monitors and other equipment, and being moved during labor.
- I wanted the baby's father to be present during birth.
- I didn't trust the hospital to let me have the baby my way.
- I dislike the use of drugs during childbirth, and I didn't trust the hospital not to give me any.

- I saw my pregnancy as a normal process, and hospitals are for sick people.
- A hospital was close by in case of emergency.
- I believe I should take responsibility for my own health.
- It costs less to have the baby at home.
- I was confident that any risks could be picked up before delivery.
- At home, I thought I'd have more control over my childbirth experience.
- I wanted my other children to be able to see the birth.
- I wanted to give birth in my own familiar surroundings.
- I thought I'd get more understanding and support during my birth at home. People treat you too impersonally in hospitals.[2]

Preference for Hospital Birth

Still, most mothers do enter hospitals and submit to high-tech deliveries. Why? Did they deliberate the risks and benefits and thereby come to a decision? Or did they leave the thinking up to their physicians? The same researchers who polled home birth advocates also interviewed mothers who chose hospital delivery. Here is what these mothers had to say about their decision:

- I wanted the rest I would get in a hospital and wouldn't get at home.
- I was planning to be sterilized.
- The baby's father wanted me to deliver in the hospital.
- I was afraid of delivering at home in case I had a genetically abnormal baby.
- I was nervous because I hadn't had a baby in many years.
- I was nervous because this was my first baby.
- I was afraid of delivering at home because my husband works away from home a lot.
- I thought that something would go wrong if I delivered at home. It's safer to deliver in a hospital.
- I'm afraid of midwives, I don't think they know what they're doing.
- I didn't want any pain at all during labor and delivery.
- My doctor wouldn't deliver me out of the hospital.
- I trust my doctor, and he thought I should deliver in the hospital.

- There was a good chance I'd have complications during delivery, and I had to deliver in the hospital.
- I developed complications during pregnancy and had to deliver in the hospital.
- I wanted access to all the new equipment that a hospital has.
- I wanted my baby delivered in the most modern way.[2]

The Issue of Safety

The bottom line in weighing home against hospital birth is not money or control or togetherness or atmosphere. It's safety. Are hospitals safer than homes for mothers and babies? Most people feel intuitively that they are. But when we leave the lotus land of intuition for the hard, cold world of statistics, a different picture emerges. Home birth advocates can and do point to statistics showing that homes are safer for babies as well as for mothers who are healthy and whose pregnancies have been medically uneventful. (In these statistical studies, "safety," or lack of it, means illness or death during birth or shortly thereafter.)

One survey[3] carried out at the U.S. Centers for Disease Control studied all out-of-hospital births that occurred between 1974 and 1976 in North Carolina (Table 4-1). As the table shows, it is essential, in evaluating the results of this or any other study comparing the safety of home and hospital birth, to distinguish between planned and un-

Table 4.1 Neonatal Death Rates in North Carolina, 1974–1976, by Birthplace and Birth Attendants

Birthplace	Number of Births	Birth Attendant	Neonatal Death Rate per 1000 Live Births
Hospital	242,245	Physician	12
Enroute to hospital (accidental)	949	?	16
Office or clinic	177	?	68
Home			
Planned	55	Physician	0
Planned	768	Lay midwife	4
Planned	100	Unattended	30
Unplanned	250	Unattended	120

Adapted from Burnett, C.A., and others: Home delivery and neonatal mortality in North Carolina, J.A.M.A. **244**:2741, 1980.

planned places of birth and between attended and unattended births. For example, in this study, five of the deaths following unplanned, unattended home births were suspected infanticides. (Criminal charges were actually sought against three of these mothers.) Planned, attended hospital births are appropriately compared only to planned, attended home births—not to all births.

In another study,[4] 1046 home births were compared with an equal number of hospital births. The hospital sample was matched to the home birth sample on several variables: maternal age, education, *socioeconomic status*, number of previous births, and number of *prenatal risk factors*. Among the women choosing home birth, 66% chose as their attendant the *family physician*, 31% chose a *lay-midwife*, and 3% chose a *nurse-midwife*. Among mothers choosing hospital birth, 100% were attended by an obstetrician or the family physician.

Table 4-2 shows the outcomes of this study. Although there were no statistically significant differences in infant mortality, all morbidity measures favored babies born at home. Hospital-born babies far exceeded home-born babies in respiratory distress, poor *Apgar scores*, birth injuries, neurological abnormalities, infections, and the need for resuscitation and oxygen. Forceps were used 21 times more frequently in hospital births. Mothers' data show that hospital births were characterized by heavy medication and resort to cesarean deliveries. Despite hospital reliance on episiotomy, lacerations were still substantially higher for hospitalized mothers than for mothers who chose home delivery. Postpartum hemorrhage was three times as likely following hospital birth.

The United States is not the only country with data allowing comparison of the safety of home births with that of hospital births. The Netherlands now has a population as heterogeneous as that of the United States. Nevertheless, its cesarean section rate is only 2.8%[5] (compared with almost 20% for the United States) and its infant mortality is only 60% as high as ours.[1] Why? Experts point to the Netherlands' high rate (40%) of home deliveries plus its program of careful screening for prenatal risk. A recent study considered differences among Holland's 13 largest cities in perinatal mortality and in trends toward hospital deliveries. The study's results indicate that the greatest decrease in infant deaths has occurred in cities with the highest home birth rates.[1]

It is also important to remember in home-hospital comparisons that hospitals have been shown to underreport neonatal deaths and to misrepresent the real cause of some maternal deaths. For example,

Table 4.2 Outcomes for Matched Home and Hospital Samples

	1046 Home Births	1046 Hospital Births
Babies		
Neonatal death	0	1
Respiratory distress	1	17
Resuscitation required	14	52
Oxygen required	13	93
Poor Apgar scores		
1 minute postnatal	56	116
5 minutes postnatal	11	23
Birth injuries	0	30
Forceps	17	363
Neurological abnormalities	1	6
Infection	2	8
Mothers		
Oxytocin	69	172
Analgesic drug	14	555
Anesthetic	35	803
Episiotomy	103	914
Laceration	170	223
Cesarean section	28	86
Postpartum hemorrhage	9	25

Adapted from Mehl, L.E.: Research on alternatives in childbirth. In Stewart, D., and Stewart, L., (eds.): 21st century obstetrics now!, vol. 1, Marble Hill, Mo., 1977, NAPSAC Reproductions.

Rubin and others[6] reviewed the neonatal outcome of 3369 infants who weighed less than 1500 grams who were born in Georgia between 1974 and 1976. They matched 1465 of these infants with death certificates. On reviewing hospital records for the remaining infants, they identified 453 infants whose deaths were unregistered. In a subsequent search, these researchers identified an additional 236 infants whose deaths were unregistered (40% of whom had weighed more than 1500 grams). The total represents a 21% underregistration of neonatal deaths. Georgia is not alone in underregistration of deaths of neonates born in hospitals. Underregistration of neonatal death appears to occur in most other states and to be particularly characteristic of Alaska, Florida, Idaho, South Carolina, West Virginia, and Wisconsin.[6]

Not only do hospitals underreport infant deaths but maternal deaths as well. Another group of researchers at the Centers for Disease

Control examined death certificate information for 3190 female residents of Georgia who were between 10 and 44 years of age and who died in a 26-month period beginning in 1975. The researchers then attempted to link these death certificates to certificates of live birth during a corresponding period. They found that up to 50%[6] of the death certificates failed to show that the cause of death had actually been complications of pregnancy and childbirth. The investigators point out that their figures for unreported maternal deaths are conservative in several ways. For example, their linkage was limited to women's death certificates and certificates of live births. Had they also linked women's death certificates to death certificates of *stillborn* infants, they would have found an even greater increase in the number of unreported maternal deaths.

Concealing the true extent of maternal death following hospital delivery is not limited to Georgia. Other investigators have found 28% underreporting in Minnesota, 73% in Massachusetts, 45% in New Jersey,[6] and 35.6% in Puerto Rico.[7,8] According to the Minnesota investigators, "Analysis of the maternal death certificates showed that only 35 percent were complete and correct. In 14 instances there was actual *falsification* [italics added] of the certificate. Considering the most important item of cause of death, it is seen that 70 (25%) were totally incorrect."[9]

A tragic footnote to maternal mortality statistics is that most of these deaths were preventable, in the opinions of case examiners. The National Institutes of Health, in reviewing the work of state committees on maternal mortality, concluded, "The most important finding from the investigations of these committees is that many maternal deaths are preventable."[10] For example, in Ohio, 65% of maternal deaths could have been avoided; in Rhode Island, 59%; in Mississippi, 90%; in South Carolina, 53%; in Indiana, 67%; and in California, 79%.[10] In Minnesota, out of 79 preventable maternal deaths, Barno and others attributed 69 to physicians but only one to a midwife.[9]

Why such widespread misrepresentation of maternal death statistics? Why is actual cause of death so frequently falsified by omission or commission? Because the physician who completes the death certificate is the same physician who was responsible for the dead mother's care when she was alive, and, if state committees investigating prevention are to be believed, the same physician who is often responsible for that mother's death. Like asking the accused to be his own judge and jury, it is unrealistic to expect physicians to admit their failures to themselves, to their peers, to a dead patient's family and perhaps to a lawyer. Under the circumstances, who among us would eagerly step forward and publicly proclaim "mea culpa"? It is also unrealistic to expect state maternal mortality committees to ferret out statistical inaccuracies because those committees are made up in large part, or even entirely, of obstetricians.

Finally, it is important to remember, in comparing the safety of home versus hospital delivery, that there are an unknown number of healthy babies whose home births are never registered. If one considers these, together with the underreporting of mother and infant deaths, the safety in favor of home births becomes even greater.

Maternal (as well as infant) mortality statistics compiled by the National Center for Health Statistics are generally regarded as definitive for the United States. Nevertheless, since they are based on state statistics, they also are correspondingly biased in painting a too rosy picture of safety for hospital delivery. After comparing maternal mortality at the state and national levels, one researcher concluded that statistical underreporting at the national level is as high as 50%.[6]

5

Your Decision

Responsibility and Control

Parenthood is forever. Most parents cannot, under the ground rules of our society, decide that their baby is not up to expectations and leave it in the hospital nursery when they leave for home, as they could leave a defective piece of merchandise at the store. Nor will the obstetrician accept responsibility for the baby, even if he or she is at fault for its being less than perfect. The medical model stresses authority, not responsibility. So no matter what happens to the baby at the hospital, it is still the parents' responsibility—physically, financially, and psychologically. And this responsibility continues every minute of every day for the next 20 years or more. You may divorce your spouse in those two decades, but you may not divorce your children.

This is a responsibility of the most mind-boggling dimensions. It demands a proportionate amount of authority and control. In other words, because the burden of responsibility is all yours, you must also have the authority to make decisions affecting that responsibility. Looking at it from a different perspective, neither you nor your baby can afford to relinquish decision-making authority to someone who will not shoulder future responsibility for those decisions.

Unfortunately, neither doctors nor hospital staff acknowledge this fundamental balance between present decision-making control and ultimate responsibility. Instead, physicians take all of the control but none of the responsibility. As one concerned physician remarked, "The great arrogance of the physician is . . . in his expropriation of the dearest right of life, the right to control one's own destiny."[1] Another commented:

> The ... most important issue is that of control. At the very time that a young couple are about to become a family, that they are on the verge of taking on the awesome responsibility of parenthood, at a time when everything should be done to bolster their self-esteem and sense of autonomy and personal responsibility, all decisions are taken out of their hands. When it is most important that they learn to function as adults, they are treated like children. So-called experts tell them what to do and brook no interference.

> I recently heard of a young couple who were told by the doctor that she was to come into the hospital the next day for an induction. Her pregnancy had been perfectly normal, and the only reason given was that she was 10 days overdue. When the doctor was asked to explain why the induction was necessary, he simply replied that he was in charge, and that if she didn't come in for the induction, she could find another obstetrician. He would no longer look after her.[2]

This issue of control is uppermost in this excerpt from a letter of complaint written by a mother to her obstetrician.

> When my husband questioned you, you snapped at him and said that you would not stand for having your medical judgment questioned and that you were in charge and that if he didn't like it he/we could leave. First: He and I have every right to question you. You are not God. You are a human doctor who we are paying a great deal of money to assist in the delivery of our child. You are there to offer medical judgment and perform medical services, not to give us orders.

> ... Further, saying that we could leave if we didn't do things your way is a really cheap trick. On a cold day it is not practical for a woman with ruptured membranes, partially dilated, to put on wet clothes and go out looking for a new obstetrician. That smacks of extortion.

> ... All in all, I feel that you allowed your personal desire to play God to interfere with your medical judgment and made the birth of my third child less joyful than it should have been.

Information and Decision Making

Competent decision making requires information on which to base that decision. Research consistently indicates that health care consumers want information about health-related matters, that they use such information competently, and that providing information to them has positive consequences for their mental as well as physical health.

Most health care agencies and professional groups are publicly committed to the policy of providing information to consumers.[3] For example, the American Medical Association, the American Academy of Pediatrics, the American College of Obstetricians and Gynecologists, the American Hospital Association, the American Society of Hospital Pharmacists, the Federal Trade Commission, the Food and Drug Administration (FDA), and the Office of Technology Assessment have all publicly pledged to provide consumers with information. In practice, however, these groups are not generous with consumer information. Sometimes they purposely withhold important consumer information. For example, in 1979, the FDA's Advisory Committee on Anesthetic and Life Support Drugs unanimously conceded that obstetrical drugs produce adverse effects in neonates. The committee then voted to withhold this information from physicians and from parents of the 7 million infants who are annually affected by the drugs.

In September, 1982, another anticonsumer move came to light. Citing a Reagan-reduced budget, the FDA vetoed a consumer-proposed program to require informational brochures called "patient package inserts" to be dispensed along with some frequently used prescription drugs.[4]

Physicians do not dispense information more generously or accurately to individual patients than to the general public. As one mother wrote her obstetrician following the birth of her third child,

> When we questioned you further (about the advisability of induction), you said that induction was risk free. The risks include cerebral hemorrhage and ruptured uterus. The risks may be slight, but I have the right to a truthful explanation to exactly what those risks are. It is after all not you who are taking the risk, but me and my child.

How do mothers who choose hospital birth fare with respect to information and control over their own pregnancies and deliveries? A team of researchers recently conducted a study of 602 mothers, some of whom had chosen traditional, in-hospital delivery and some of whom had chosen out-of-hospital delivery either at a freestanding birth center or at home. The purpose of the study was to investigate drug consumption during pregnancy and childbirth, the status of those drugs with respect to safety for the baby, and the amount of information mothers have about the drugs to which their babies are thus exposed.

Results showed that during pregnancy as well as childbirth, mothers choosing traditional delivery consumed significantly more prescription drugs, nonprescription drugs, and druglike products than mothers choosing nontraditional delivery. Further, for mothers delivering in-hospital, there was no relationship between prenatal drug consumption and the number of drugs administered by medical personnel during labor and delivery, suggesting that women choosing traditional delivery forfeit decision-making control when they enter the hospital. Few drugs used in hospital deliveries were clearly safe for babies.

Mothers also differed in terms of the amount of information they had about the drugs they consumed and to which their babies were exposed. Mothers birthing at home had twice as much drug information as mothers delivering in-hospital. Those mothers with the highest drug information scores consumed the fewest drugs. Why did so many mothers have so little information about drugs? Although their obstetricians were generous in prescribing drugs, they were miserly in dispensing information about those drugs to their pregnant patients. To share information is to share power, and most physicians are unwilling to do that.

There was another startling contrast among the three groups of mothers. Psychological tests revealed that nontraditionally delivered mothers perceived themselves in control of their environments, whereas traditionally delivered mothers perceived that the environment controlled them.

No Information, No Control: Consequences for Consumers

As we have seen, information is an essential part of the perception that one is able to control one's own life. Several studies have dealt with the consequences of providing or withholding information about health-related matters. They may be summarized as follows:

Consequences of providing information to patients about their conditions and about the indicated therapy for those conditions. Several investigations have studied the effects of providing information to patient-consumers about their conditions and about indicated therapy for those conditions. The effects are consistently positive. They include reports of decreased pain, decreased need for narcotics and other drugs, more effective coping with the medical condition, faster physical recovery, decreased length of hospitalization, increased compliance, and improved morale, as well as greater satisfaction with the health care provided.

Consequences of withholding information and of perceived loss of control over events relating to one's own health. The outcomes of these studies are consistent in demonstrating negative consequences of withholding information. Demonstrated emotional consequences include anger, anxiety, and depression, as well as psychological withdrawal. Cognitive and behavioral consequences include decreased ability to take in and to disclose information about one's own health to health care professionals ("cognitive neglect"); decreased ability to process new information objectively and validly ("cognitive immobilization"); indiscriminate demands for health-related information; decreased compliance; and increased complaints, apathy, extreme passivity, or learned helplessness, including decreased abilities to learn and to cope with one's environment. Physiological consequences include increased reported pain; increased number of reported symptoms; increased morbidity and hypertension; elevated catecholamine excretion, followed by adrenaline depletion and high levels of hydrocortisone.[3]

Getting Information
Use the Library

Even when physicians may base their decisions on blind faith, uncritical acceptance of authority, or other nonscientific factors, it is not necessary for you to do so. You can make your own evaluation, starting at the nearest medical library. As Mendelsohn noted in his *Confessions of a Medical Heretic*, "Anybody with an eighth grade education and a dictionary can read any medical book."[6] Said another consumer advocate, "Truly informed consent . . . can be achieved in most situations in direct proportion to the effort a consumer is willing to expend in self-education."[7]

The first step in getting enough accurate information on which to base a decision is to review the published evidence bearing on benefits and risks of the various obstetrical interventions. Medical literature is available to you in the medical school libraries of public universities. (In considering this, remember that your tax dollars support public institutions.[8]) If you need help, ask the reference librarian, whose job it is to show you where things are and how to use the library. The interlibrary loan librarian can also assist by borrowing from other libraries those items not owned by your own medical library. In addition, you may wish to ask the Medline librarian to help in using the computerized medical literature search and retrieval system. This time-saving system prints out references to all recent literature on a particular subject, for example, circumcision or cesarean section. It is like an electronic research assistant. There may be a charge for use of the Medline computer.[12] If you are short on money but long on time, it is possible to get the same set of references on any subject by using *Index Medicus*. The reference librarian can show you where this is and how to use it.[13]

If all this seems like a lot of extra work, remember that you owe it to yourself and your unborn baby to be well informed and accurately informed.

Look at Films

Books are invaluable sources of information. Still, such an active event as birthing is hard to convey in words. As the old saying goes, one picture is worth a thousand words. Every pregnant woman is naturally curious to see how birth happens, how much apparent discomfort is involved, what transpires between her and her birth attendants, and what happens to the baby.

Fortunately, there are lots of childbirth films available: birth in the hospital (including cesarean birth), birth at home, birth at a freestanding birth center, birth from a consumer's point of view, and so on. (See Appendix B for an annotated list of childbirth films.) Unfortunately, most of these movies are commercially made and are distributed only to those who can afford to rent them. Rental fees for films available through the Filmakers Library[14] catalog range from $20 to $40, averaging about $35 for a single showing. Rental fees for films available from university audiovisual departments are less, averaging about $15 for a 2-day rental period.

It is of course possible to share movie rental fees with other pregnant women, which means joining an organized group or organizing your own. The organized groups most readily found in towns or cities of any size are childbirth education classes. However, childbirth education class teachers typically have an established teaching agenda that may not be very flexible or easy to modify. If you live in a town or city of reasonable size, you may find other groups that have organized themselves around change-oriented childbirth groups, freestanding birth centers, women's health centers, or other consumer-oriented agencies.

Another possibility is to locate video exchange retailers who stock, or are willing to stock, childbirth films among the more traditional films in their inventories. Video exchange retailers rent films recorded on video cassette tapes to owners of home video recorders. Their rental fees are as low as $2 per night.[15]

Talk with Other Mothers

Even though the scientific literature may be nonexistent with respect to emotional and psychological risks of intervention procedures, it is possible for you to do your own "research" by talking with experienced mothers. Mothers delight in describing their birth experiences to interested listeners, particularly mothers-to-be. Interview several, making sure to include mothers who have given birth at home, mothers who have given birth in a freestanding birth center, and mothers who have given birth in hospitals. If you can find mothers who have given birth in two different places—hospital and home or hospital and birth center— so much the better for comparison purposes.

If you can find just one mother who has given birth in a hospital and another who has given birth at home, they will probably be able to put you in touch with other mothers who have given birth in the same places. However, if you are a stranger in town or don't know any mothers, ask a childbirth or breastfeeding group for help in locating mothers you can interview. Childbirth educators both in the Bradley and the Lamaze methods can help you locate mothers who have given birth in the hospital as well as in the home. There may also be childbirth educators in your area specializing in instruction for home birth who are certified by Home Oriented Maternity Experience (HOME), Association for Childbirth at Home International (ACHI), or Informed Homebirth, Inc. (see Appendix C).

Because they must issue birth certificates, the medical records department of the county in which you reside has the names of all the county residents who have given birth there. You can also obtain a copy of the International Association of Parents and Professionals for Safe Alternatives in Childbirth (NAPSAC) Directory of Alternative Birth Services (see Appendix C), which contains thousands of names of midwives, home birth programs, birth centers, natural childbirth doctors, and family-centered hospitals.

After you locate a mother, you're ready to talk with her. Ask her what she liked about her birth experience and what she disliked. Ask her about each of the intervention procedures mentioned in this book. Ask her where and how she will choose to have her next baby. See Appendix B for published reports comparing home and hospital as places of birth.

Determine Your Risk Status

The concept of medical risk was discussed in Chapter 1. In this context, "risk" means the probability that delivery will be normal ("uneventful," in medical jargon) or beset by one or more complications. This probability is the end result of inventorying the health-related problems that predispose toward delivery complications. If you have no health problems, yours is a low-risk pregnancy; if many health problems, a high-risk pregnancy. Most out-of-hospital birth attendants accept only mothers whose pregnancies are low risk.

There is nothing magic about inventorying health. You can do it yourself, possibly with the help of a doctor or midwife who has had experience with out-of-hospital births. The major factors associated with delivery risk are these:

- Complications of your present pregnancy, including *hypertension*, toxemia, preeclampsia or *eclampsia*, *placenta previa*, more than one fetus, fetal position other than head first, *cord prolapse*.
- Complications in previous pregnancies, including cesarean section, hemorrhage, prematurity, stillbirth, three or more miscarriages.
- Current health problems, including venereal disease, drug addiction, mental illness, heart or kidney disease, epilepsy, or other serious medical conditions.
- No prenatal care for the first two trimesters of current pregnancy.
- Six or more previous births.
- More than 40 years of age (if multiparous) or 36 years of age (if primiparous).

Should it be necessary to inventory your risk status after your child's birth rather than before, a disgruntled mother suggests some ground rules:

Despite all my precautions, I recently was victimized by an unnecessary cesarean. After much soul searching, I decided to turn some of my anger and frustration back at the medical profession to see if I could get any satisfaction.

First, I obtained my hospital records. The clerk at the hospital didn't want to let me see them, but when I said I had a right to see them and I was prepared to call my lawyer, I was given them at 75 cents per page copying fee. I studied the records and came up with many questions about what they said, which I wrote down. For example, there was discrepancy about what my doctor told me regarding my failure to progress at a time the nurse's notes said I had gone from four to five cms. dilation.

I also did some research about cesareans. I read *Williams' Obstetrics,* the National Institutes of Health report on cesareans, C/SEC's information packet, and the book *Birthing Normally.* These raised further questions about the basis for my obstetrician's diagnosis. I wrote these down too.

I also learned about alternatives to surgery which ranged from drugs to just plain time and emotional support, which I would have expected my doctor (who represented himself as knowledgeable on natural childbirth) to know. In addition, I got several medical opinions regarding the necessity of my own cesarean. Besides reviewing my labor with my husband, labor coaches, midwives, and childbirth educators, I also made appointments with two other physicians who read my records. Both of them felt my cesarean was not medically indicated at the time it was done.

After thus learning all I could about my cesarean and cesareans in general, I consulted several lawyers about the possibility of suit. The consensus was that the suit would be uneconomic because my damages were largely emotional and temporary (loss of a natural birth experience), which society does not yet consider worth much.

I then decided that the best course for me would be to write a confidential letter to the obstetrician with a copy and confidential cover letter to the medical director of the hospital. I wrote the strongest possible letter, expressing my feelings and raising some of the many questions I had, and requested a hearing. I was given one and I did receive some amount of satisfaction—if not a better understanding of what had happened, then at least the knowledge that my doctor realized how strongly I felt about what he had done.

Based on my own experience with the hearing, I would stress for other people the importance of: (1) being prepared when you go, (2) acting in confidence and being truthful (never backing down on your feelings), (3) being respectful to the doctor (never calling him names), and (4) bringing someone with you to act as a witness of what transpires.

If I felt my hearing was not fruitful, I would have done any number of
other things, which I would like to present to you now:
- Going to the regular hospital board with a strong letter of
  complaint and request for hearing.
- Going to the county medical society with same.
- Asking for a government audit to determine if unnecessary
  surgery is being done. (This would apply if the hospital received government funds.)
- Working to obtain the exact cesarean statistics and trying to
  get them publicized in the newspaper, either directly or by
  testifying at public hearings such as on the hospital's ac-
  creditation. (These hearings don't come up too often, so
  your timing would have to be right.)
- Going to the insurance company with a complaint about
  their having to foot the bill for so much unnecessary surgery.
- Demanding that the hospital give the money back for the
  surgery, the hospital stay, or both. If I had realized it earlier
  I could have refused to pay the bill, with the onus on them
  to try and collect. (A hospital can't hold you prisoner over
  money once you've been medically released. See Annas, G.:
  The rights of hospital patients, New York, 1975, Avon
  Books.)
- Taking the case to small claims court to make a point.
  (Check what the monetary limit is in your state.)
- Writing letters to the hospital's board of directors.
- Organizing a demonstration at the hospital with picket-
  ing.[17]

Estimate the Cost of Delivery

A hospital delivery costs more than a freestanding birth center delivery and much more than a home delivery. In addition, the cost of hospital delivery depends on the region in which you live. New York City is
more expensive than Morgantown, West Virginia. Finally, the cost of
delivery depends on your insurance coverage. Few insurance companies have extended coverage to home births, although some cover
births in freestanding birth centers. Coverage of hospital births varies
depending on the source of insurance, the length of time you have held
the policy, and so forth.

Because your financial situation is unique, it will be necessary for
you to do your own research here as well. If you're planning a hospital
birth, ask the director of the accounts or billing department of that
hospital about the daily room rates for youself, as well as nursery rates

for babies. (Remember that you and the baby will have to stay several more days if you have a cesarean delivery.) Ask also about the following: charge for use of electronic fetal monitor, ultrasound, labor room charges, delivery room charges, operating room charges (in case of cesarean section), and anesthetist charges, including whether you must pay an anesthetist if you don't use anesthesia.

• • •

Remember that retaining control through decision making requires getting the information necessary for making those decisions. By medical tradition, obstetrical patients retain responsibility but relinquish control over decisions that vitally effect them and their babies. Thus does inequity generate iniquity.

6

Legal Aspects of Childbirth

Giving birth is not something most people think about in a legal context. Until the early 1940s most women gave birth at home, and it was considered to be a significant social and medical advancement when labor and delivery were moved to a hospital setting. The move to hospitals put childbirth into a more "scientific" arena, and before long giving birth became a medical process involving numerous drug and instrument interventions.

Only recently has there been information available indicating that medical-technical intervention in the birthing process may actually be harmful. Because women have become more aware of health and psychological factors associated with pregnancy and childbirth, there has been a substantial movement to reverse the technical trend and return to a more natural and uninhibited birthing process.

Women no longer necessarily fill the role of mother and homemaker. They are deciding when to have a child, and the decision is often a result of much planning. There is unquestionably an increasing awareness of the physiological as well as psychological aspects of birth. Today's women have heard many unhappy stories from their mothers and friends about hospital experiences of childbirth, such as attendance by insensitive doctors and hospital personnel; use of degrading, uncomfortable, and sometimes harmful procedures for the convenience of staff rather than for the benefit of mother and child; interference with bonding and breastfeeding because of hospital practices; and the use of drugs of questionable safety or efficacy to the infant and mother. Many persons interested in having children educate themselves fully on childbirth before conception. An array of literature is available (see Appendix B).

This chapter on various legal aspects of childbirth is not meant to be comprehensive but to give you information about how you might be affected by the law, how you might use the law to make your own decisions relating to childbirth, and how you might participate in bringing about necessary changes in current hospital practices in obstetrics. Some general questions will be answered, but specific problems should be referred to a person trained in the law. Your selection of a lawyer is as important as the selection of your physician or midwife.

There are some general legal principles that apply to all states, but many of the concepts discussed in the following chapters are not settled areas of the law. George Annas, author of numerous books dealing with patient rights, sums up the legal aspects of childbirth: (1) the law is very conservative, (2) the law varies from state to state, and (3) the law is outcome oriented.[1] It is useful to hire a lawyer who shares an interest in your case. You may have access to a law library, a legal aid society, or an activist women's organization that can help you find the right attorney. Organizations established to aid women who have received inappropriate or negligent health care include the Alternative Birth Crisis Coalition (see Appendix C) and the Litigation Information Service, set up by the National Women's Health Network.[2]

An initial recommendation is to read as much as possible in the areas of pregnancy, labor, and delivery and discuss these topics with knowledgeable friends and professionals. Find out if there are any women's health groups that can provide information on the various birthing alternatives in your community. If you are lucky, you will learn of childbearing facilities that are consistent with your educated decision about the type of birth you want for yourself and your child. If not, you may want to join the thousands of prospective parents who are insisting that they have a voice in their fundamental procreative rights.

Means of Controlling the Birthing Experience
Choice of Setting and Professionals

Two of the most important decisions you will ever make are choosing where you will give birth and who is to assist you. Most communities offer a variety of possibilities, including home birth with midwife assistance, home-oriented birthing centers with professional attendants, birthing rooms situated in the obstetrical sections of hospitals that allow for natural and uninterrupted labor and delivery, and the typical obstetrics ward of a hospital with its attendant standardized procedures (as described in Chapter 1) that are considered to be accepted practices in the medical community.

In choosing a birth setting and birth attendant, it is important to consider not only your legal rights but also those of the developing child. There is continuing controversy concerning the legal rights of the fetus. Courts have historically declined to impose a legal duty on a woman to provide care to the child during the time of birth,[3] though more recent cases find *liability* where the *negligence* has been gross.[4] It is generally conceded that a *viable* fetus has rights that must be balanced against the mother's rights in the area of abortion law[5] and in laws relating to birth to the extent that states may require the licensing of persons who assist others in birth.[6] Although women have a "right to privacy" with respect to contraception and previability abortion, "the right to privacy has never been interpreted so broadly as to protect a woman's choice of the manner and circumstances in which her baby is to be born."[6] And although a majority of states do not consider a fetus a "person" for the purposes of bringing a *wrongful death action*, an increasing minority of jurisdictions now allow this,[7] indicating an expansion of fetal rights. California still does not allow a fetus to bring a wrongful death action,[8] and a California court dismissed charges of felonious child-endangering against the mother whose twin sons were born addicted to heroin and suffering withdrawal.[9]

A court was willing to intercede on behalf of a fetus in Georgia when the Department of Human Resources petitioned the court for temporary custody of an unborn child because the parents had refused for religious reasons to consent to a cesarean operation. The mother had suffered a complete placenta previa (that is, the afterbirth was between the baby and the birth canal), and the physicians predicted with 99% certainty that the child could not survive a vaginal delivery. Temporary custody of the unborn was given to the department, and the court ordered the mother to submit to a *sonogram*, cesarean section, and related procedures for the benefit of the unborn child. The parents' *motion for a stay* of the *lower court's* order was denied by the Georgia Supreme Court.[10] This case was concluded happily. The complications apparently corrected themselves, and the mother had an uneventful vaginal delivery, without the assistance of the Georgia Department of Human Resources. However, a Colorado woman was ordered to undergo a cesarean section against her wishes by a judge presiding in her labor room. In that case, doctors had recommended a cesarean delivery because of *meconium* staining in the amniotic fluid, abnormal fetal heart tracings, and a high presenting part. When the mother refused, the legal staff of the hospital petitioned the juvenile court to find the unborn child "dependent" and therefore under the jurisdiction of the court so that the judge could then order the cesarean because it was in the best interest of the child.[11] The mother's interests and desires were considered secondary. Other courts have held that treatment of the mother can be ordered to protect the rights of the unborn fetus.[12] These cases raise important questions concerning the right of governmental authorities to intervene in fundamentally private matters and illustrate an increasing willingness to do so.[13]

Home Birth Assisted by Midwives

Midwifery has been defined as "the furthering or undertaking by any person to assist a woman in normal childbirth."[6] Before the 1940s, it was not unusual for certain segments of the population, generally the rural poor, to have their births attended by untrained persons. Most states distinguish between lay-midwives and certified nurse-midwives both in terms of responsibility and liability. A lay- or *empirical-midwife* has no formal certification and often does not have any professional training. Some states require licensing, and some limit the practice only when money is involved. In other words, there is no prohibition against lay assistance in childbirth if the attendant does not charge a fee. No state requires a woman to have her child in a hospital or forbids home birth. A woman may legally deliver a child unattended or assisted only by her husband. In this situation, the only possible legal ramification might be if there is extreme neglect or unconscionable disregard for the well-being of the fetus or child.

A certified nurse-midwife is a person educated at the professional level in both nursing and midwifery. There are about 21 nurse-midwifery programs in the United States that have been approved by the American College of Nurse-Midwives. They prepare individuals already trained as registered nurses to care for the health needs of healthy women and their infants during pregnancy, labor, delivery, and the postpartum period. Nurse-midwives must pass a national, written certification examination in addition to completing an approved educational program to use the designation of "certified nurse-midwife."

The medical profession has often opposed the expansion of midwife services, regardless of the qualifications. In California, for example, a Professional Midwifery Practice Act was first introduced in the legislature in 1977. Proponents of the bill argue that women and their families have the right to safe alternatives in obstetrical care. Strong opposition has come from the California Medical Association, and the bill has not yet been enacted into law.[14] Existing midwife provisions in several states are useless because they require that midwives be supervised by physicians. However, physicians have an economic conflict of interest and either refuse to supervise midwives or else set up requirements that are impossible for midwives to meet.

Consumer demands for alternative birth plans have clashed head on with serious pressure from the medical profession against such alternatives. Opposition from the medical community may be directly related to economic rather than safety factors, since there has not been the same sort of opposition when midwives care for poor women who are unable to pay for services or who are uninsured.[15] In addition, statistics that compare complication rates for trained midwife-assisted births with hospital births show that the midwife-assisted birth is safer.[16]

Examples of the type of pressure being exerted against the expansion of midwifery include civil and criminal suits against practicing midwives, refusal of physician-controlled boards to grant midwives licenses, restraint of trade through restricting or revoking hospital privileges, difficulties in arranging for alternative delivery when complications arise, refusal of insurance companies to authorize payment to midwives, opposition from pediatricians, and conspiracy of doctors against doctors who participate in alternative birth plans. Each of these will be briefly discussed.

Civil and criminal suits against practicing midwives. In 1979 a practicing lay-midwife in Florida was criminally charged with the unlawful practice of medicine, and a civil injunction was sought to prevent her from continuing her practice. These suits were initiated because of the complaints of a physician. There were no complaints from the clients of the midwife. Ultimately, criminal charges were abandoned. After the trial, the court granted a motion to dismiss the civil injunction because of a finding that the statute licensing midwives gave unconstitutional discretion to the licensing authority without sufficient legislative guidelines and because the law was vague.[17] It was not until 1982 that the Florida legislature adopted a new statute that provided for the licensing of midwives in accordance with stipulated, legislative guidelines.[18]

In California in 1974 state undercover agents made arrangements for two unlicensed midwives to come to a fake birth and then arrested them on the criminal charge of practicing a healing art without a license.[6] Attorneys for the midwives challenged the constitutionality of the statute, asserting, among other things, that it violated a mother's right to privacy and that pregnancy is a normal condition, not a sickness or affliction as defined by the statute. The court upheld the statute, finding that the state has a recognized interest in the life and well-being of an unborn child and in the requirement for the licensing of midwives. The court, in its opinion, recommended that the arguments on the safety of home deliveries be addressed to the legislature.

In 1977 a lay-midwife in California was charged with the murder of an infant and other felonies relating to her practice of midwifery. The infant died several hours after the midwife assisted at the birth. The midwife had previously assisted in over 350 births without a single fatality. The labor and delivery were normal, but the child did not appear to be breathing on birth and was immediately transferred to a hospital. Although the murder charge was dismissed before the trial, the case proceeded to trial on counts of practicing medicine without a license and grand theft (for charging for her services). At trial, a world-renowned expert in infant pathology testified that when the baby arrived at the hospital, it was alive and capable of being resuscitated but that the hospital resuscitation team had pumped air into the baby's trachea at too high a pressure, causing its death.[19] The midwife was ultimately exonerated of all charges except one misdemeanor count of practicing medicine without a license. She received a 1-year suspended jail sentence with the condition that she not attend, even as a coach, any births for 2 years.

Refusal of physician-controlled boards to grant midwives licenses. Ten states currently allow lay midwives to practice (Arizona, Delaware, Florida, Maryland, Minnesota, Mississippi, New Mexico, Tennessee, Texas, and Washington). Some states have midwife-licensing procedures, but the licensing boards refuse to approve any licensing or they set up guidelines that are impossible to meet. For example, in Florida, only a few lay-midwife licenses have been granted in the last 15 years although there has been a midwife licensing statute on the books since 1931. It is estimated that there are several hundred actively practicing unlicensed midwives. A new statute was passed in 1982 with a stated legislative purpose of providing alternatives in birthing practices. This statute requires for licensing attendance at a state-approved school, which has not yet been established.

In North Carolina, the state agency has refused to issue any lay-midwife licenses in over 16 years.[20] An effort was made in North Carolina to bring a class action suit against the state licensing board on behalf of lay-midwives denied the right to practice midwifery and on behalf of consumers denied their services. However, this suit was not brought because the *plaintiffs* did not have the money to pay for the legal fees.[20] The refusal of the agency to set up reasonable licensing criteria is arguably an *unconstitutional restraint on trade* and a violation of civil rights. The filing of such an action might result in the establishment of reasonable licensing criteria.

Restraint of trade through restricting or revoking hospital privileges. There is considerable resistance on the part of physicians, hospitals, and medical boards to grant hospital privileges to midwives, even with the requirement that they work in conjunction with medical doctors. Some of the reasons offered include fear of diminished quality in patient care, economic competition, and malpractice claims. There is substantial evidence that combined physician-midwifery services are highly successful,[21] leaving one to conclude that much of the objection to hospital privileges for midwives is based on economic factors.

Suits have been filed challenging medical doctors' monopoly of hospital delivery rooms. An antitrust suit was filed by two certified nurse-midwives in Tennessee who attempted to set up a hospital nurse-midwifery practice. Although they had a physician willing to back them up, they were unable to obtain hospital privileges at any area hospital. In addition, the cooperative physician subsequently had his liability insurance canceled. This case is pending. A similar suit was filed in Ohio in 1981. Since that suit was filed, a Hospital Licensure Bill was passed in Ohio, which prevents anyone but doctors from admitting patients to hospitals. Efforts are currently under way to fight for the repeal of this law.

Difficulties in arranging for alternate delivery when complications arise. If you are planning a home delivery that does not involve the supervision of a physician affiliated with a hospital, you must make advance arrangements for hospitalization should that become necessary. Without such an arrangement, the hospital may not be required to accept you as a patient except under emergency conditions. Furthermore, the hospital may not regard the imminent delivery of a child as an emergency. In Mississippi, a woman went into labor more than a week earlier than expected. She was denied admission at the closest available hospital even though she was having contractions every 5 minutes. She was told to go to another hospital some 30 miles away where she had received prenatal care. The woman gave birth in a car in the hospital parking lot. After the birth, the hospital refused to admit the woman and her newborn child. The court denied relief in an action against the hospital, finding that the hospital regulations requiring a referral by local physicians, except in a true emergency, were reasonable.[22] Also, doctors who fear malpractice might refuse to get involved if, in their opinion, the labor has already been mismanaged.

Refusal of insurance companies to authorize payment to midwives. Another serious interference in the right to select alternative birth styles is the refusal, in many cases, of insurance companies to authorize payment to certified or licensed midwives who assist in home births. There are no known insurance provisions to reimburse unlicensed lay-midwives. The usual arrangement for midwife payment is for the insurance company to pay the attending physician who then pays the midwife. Some states have passed legislation providing for direct payment of nurse-midwives, but this is not true in most states. In Florida, for example, Blue Cross/Blue Shield will now directly reimburse licensed midwives. Pennsylvania and New York now also permit the direct reimbursement of nurse-midwives working under qualified medical direction and practicing in conjunction with a hospital or clinic. The American College of Obstetricians and Gynecologists approves reimbursement to midwives if services are rendered by a member of a health care team directed by a qualified obstetrician.[23] Even though the costs associated with midwife-assisted childbirth are generally much lower than hospital births, many women cannot afford a midwife's services because of lack of insurance coverage.

Since 1982, the United States government, through Medicaid, allows nurse-midwives to be paid as independent practitioners whether or not they work under the supervision of a physician.[23a] Military dependents and retirees are also covered for midwifery services under the Civilian Health and Medical Program of the Uniformed Services (CHAMPUS).

Opposition from pediatricians. In some areas the local medical community has such opposition to home births that it is difficult to find a pediatrician to examine the child shortly after birth. The American Academy of Pediatrics has taken a formal position against home deliveries for all women.[24] It is recommended that a woman arrange for the services of a pediatrician before the child's birth regardless of where the birth takes place. This is particularly important if a home birth is planned. The pediatrician should be committed in writing to attend the child after birth.

Conspiracy of doctors against doctors who participate in alternative birth plans. Not all physicians oppose alternatives to hospital births. Some have cooperated in supervising midwife programs, in and out of hospital settings. Frequently, this kind of cooperation results in sanctions imposed by the medical profession against the cooperating physician. For example, a physician who operated a birth center and home birth service in Oklahoma City lost his malpractice insurance in January, 1981, because of his involvement with out-of-hospital births. Other doctors in the community refused to provide back-up support.[25] Another obstetrician in Nashville, Tennessee, lost his malpractice insurance in 1980 because he served as a back-up to a hospital-based nurse-midwifery service. The insurance company denied coverage because of an alleged increased risk, and the physician was ostracized by other area doctors.[25] The licensed nurse-midwives who were attempting to set up a hospital-based midwifery practice in Nashville have been unable to obtain the cooperation of a single hospital in the area. This controversy led to a congressional hearing in December 1980 to investigate whether there existed an unfair restraint of trade against the midwives.[15] It also led to the civil suit mentioned earlier.

Hospital Birth

Selecting hospital and physician. If you choose an in-hospital birth, it is important to select the physician and the hospital. Procedures vary from hospital to hospital. A physician is somewhat bound by the practices and procedures of the hospital. The obstetrician you hire to deliver your baby may not, in fact, be available the moment you go into labor. You should find out what the chances are of this occurring and also what arrangements will be made in case your physician does not happen to be available when you begin labor. It is also important for you to discuss the philosophy of childbirth with your physician. If you want to have a natural birth, you will want to know as much as possible about your physician and the hospital.

Hospitals and physicians vary considerably in cesarean section rates, that is, rates of surgical delivery. These differences in rates reflect differences in attitudes about childbirth. Some physicians simply think it is easier to perform cesarean deliveries. A concern for malpractice suits causes some physicians to allow labor to progress only a few hours before intervening, even though the first stage of labor for *primiparas* normally averages 12 to 15 hours.[26]

If the hospital requires you to pay for an anesthetist even if you've stated a preference for a drug-free delivery, the services will likely be used. Some hospitals require fetal monitoring and IVs.

Many hospitals are now accommodating the move toward more natural births by providing birthing rooms within the obstetrical wards. If so, find out how many laboring mothers can be accommodated in this way and about your chances of having access to this facility on your anticipated due date. Some physicians are willing to abide by a woman's stated desires even if they differ from procedures commonly used by hospital staff, such as pubic shaving, enemas, and supine position for labor. *Newsweek* recently reported the "discovery" of vertical delivery by modern-thinking doctors in New York. A few doctors have noticed that because of the structure of the human pelvis, "delivering a baby is best and most naturally done in a sitting or squatting position."[27] Try to reach an agreement with the doctor before you begin labor, because when labor has begun, it will be much more difficult to enforce your wishes if they differ from those of the doctor or hospital.

A Patient's Bill of Rights was affirmed by the Board of Trustees of the American Hospital Association in 1972. It is reprinted in full in Appendix G. Unfortunately, this statement has no enforcement clause and fewer than half the AHA-member hospitals have formally adopted it.[28] Hospitals vary considerably on recognition of patients' rights during delivery.

Whether a father (or significant other) is allowed in the delivery room is a policy decision that has been the source of legal controversy. Parents often feel that the birth of their child is an event to be shared and one that has tremendous psychological implications for all members of the family. Also, the laboring woman derives confidence and support from another's presence. A supportive person in the delivery room can help the laboring mother assert her desires with respect to labor management and can maintain an accurate history of the labor, including medications used and whether or not consent was obtained for medication and procedures.

In several instances, prospective parents have tried to force changes in hospital procedures through suits for injunctive relief. Several legal theories have been forwarded in these suits. When the hospital is a public facility or private but receiving government assistance, plaintiffs have stated that constitutional rights have been infringed by hospital policy, such as the mother's right to privacy. Courts have been very reluctant to interfere with the internal operating procedures of hospitals. Only a few courts have considered challenges to obstetrical procedures, sometimes dismissing the action because of insufficient government involvement, which is required to invoke constitutional rights.[29]

In Montana, a treating obstetrician joined with the parents in seeking a court order forcing the hospital to allow the father's presence in the delivery room. An *appellate court* considered the importance of the doctor-patient relationship but found against all parties, saying that physicians must abide by rules adopted by their colleagues, even though the physician has direction over the patient.[30] The court found that the hospital rule was reasonable in light of the concerns expressed, such as increased possibility of infection, concern about malpractice suits, inadequate physical facilities that do not allow room for fathers to change their clothes without bothering the doctors, increased costs, lack of privacy for other women getting ready to deliver, strict policy concerning visitors in surgical areas favored by the state board of health, and the furtherance of harmony between physicians should the cooperating physician be absent. It is interesting that most of the concerns expressed by the hospital do not reflect the needs of the patients or psychological factors that are so important in the birthing process.

In another case, the plaintiffs alleged that the hospital's refusal to allow the father in the delivery room violated the patient's constitutional right to privacy and the doctor's right to practice medicine.[31] The federal appeals court compared obstetrical procedures to other serious hospital procedures and parents' rights to the rights of others in need of extraordinary assistance. As reluctant as courts have been to interfere with hospital operating procedures, suits of this kind have an increasing likelihood of success with the continuing accrual of scientific information showing the importance of psychological factors in childbirth, medical contraindications of procedures commonly used, and an expanding recognition of the right to privacy.

Contractual agreement with the doctor. There is no reason why a person cannot contract with a physician to define the care to be received. A *contract* is an agreement for *consideration* (usually money) between two or more people for the doing or not doing of something. The relationship between a person and a doctor is generally thought to include an element beyond a mere business arrangement because of the special requirements of the medical profession and the doctor's acceptance of the Hippocratic Oath. Doctors have a fiduciary-like obligation to their patients to look after their best interests and consider their personal needs and desires. There tends to be a special trust placed in doctors, which many foster, because of the extensive training and intimate nature of the services.

A written contract with the physician can make clear what will be done or not done. Issues that might be covered in a contract include arrangements for alternate care should the physician be unavailable for delivery; use of stirrups, fetal monitoring, enema, pubic shaving, and "routine" episiotomy; use of a birthing room, if available; choice of various techniques of producing anesthesia, if it becomes necessary; presence of the father or other coach in the delivery room; and a limitation on the presence of students or interns. (Appendix F contains a sample contract.)

On first consideration, a contract may seem a sure way of controlling the hospital birth experience. However, closer examination reveals its serious limitations. Probably the most serious is finding a physician who will sign a contract. Many doctors resent any sort of interference concerning their methods. Many doctors probably will not enter into a specific contract that does not leave certain matters up to their professional judgment. Some things that may be contracted for, such as the father's presence in the delivery room, may not present problems. Other matters, such as the use of anesthetics, induction, forceps, or cesarean delivery must, in medical opinion, be left to the judgment of the doctor as the labor progresses. Any contractual effort to manage the delivery will be so circumscribed and qualified by the doctor that it will be virtually useless in certain areas.

Nevertheless, discussing a contractual agreement with your physician will probably be very enlightening. It will reveal his or her attitudes toward many of the things that concern you as well as a willingness to treat you as a competent decision maker. Note, however, that verbal agreement may be insufficient as a binding contract, as illustrated by the following excerpts from letters received by the authors:

We (husband and wife) went in well ahead of the birth and procured from him his approval of our desires (that is, husband in delivery room, forty-five degree backrest, no drugs, Lamaze-like birth, nursing on delivery table, rooming-in, and so forth). The only demand he would not approve of was delivery in the labor room as the "hospital wouldn't allow it."

I went into labor 3 weeks early—3 cm. dilation—was not allowed to go home but told to stay. Before she was born, every demand we'd made was ignored (not allowed to walk during labor, kept flat so fractured tailbone, had to scream to get husband in delivery room). Doctor argued with me about Lamaze breathing (I'd hyperventilate, he said), paracervical and pudendal shots without asking, episiotomy, purposely cut my outer labia near urethra and stitched it up so it formed a pocket to collect urine and got infected (painful!), refused to let me nurse her on delivery table and said he'd not let me have her for 24 hours. I screamed bloody murder and got my pediatrician there. I got her about 4 hours later but wasn't allowed rooming-in as Ob/Gyn put restriction on that.

Another mother writes of contractual failure:

Contrary to what my doctor had agreed to, my husband was forced to leave me alone, I was lied to by a nurse about the purpose and effect of a medication, I was given scopolamine without my consent, I was physically assaulted and then gassed in the delivery room when I happened to come to.

We had asked for a family-centered maternity experience and our doctor had agreed to it point by point, and instead this is what we got.

And still another breach of verbal agreement (from a letter to her obstetrician):

My complaints are basically of two types: your medical judgment and your attitude . . . . I came to you because you and your partner claimed to be advocates of natural childbirth. I asked if I could do a Leboyer style delivery, to which you readily agreed, as long as the baby was not to be immersed in water, a condition I found acceptable and justifiable. It was also agreed that my husband would be present throughout labor and delivery.

My water broke at about midnight. I went to the hospital as instructed and throughout the night nothing much happened. The next morning about 9:00 you breezed in and examined me. After the exam you turned to the nurse and said "pit her," and started to walk out. My husband asked for an explanation. You told him I would be induced and when he questioned you about the feasibility of waiting to see if something happened, you snapped at him and said that you would not stand for having your medical judgment questioned and that you were in charge and that if he didn't like it he/we could leave.

Contractual agreement with the hospital. When you register with a hospital, you are required to sign an agreement (perhaps several) that involves payment for services and various procedures used by the hospital. You should read carefully any agreement you sign and make sure you understand what it means. Request and keep a copy of the agreement. (See sample hospital agreement in Appendix J.) The hospital agreement may subject you to procedures you do not want.

One of the issues in a New York case was the failure of the hospital to obtain the mother's consent to a resident's delivering the baby under the supervision of the attending physician. It was the custom of that hospital for all obstetricians to allow residents in training to do complicated deliveries. The court held that by going to that particular hospital, the woman consented to the customs and practices of that hospital.[32]

Written agreements are often required when a father or coach is allowed in the delivery room. Some of the provisions might include the following: consent of the mother and attending physician, completion of childbirth education classes, scrubbing and wearing hospital garb, an agreement that the obstetrician will have the final word concerning the presence of others in the delivery room, and specific provisions relating to the use of cameras and tape recorders.

After you have gone into labor is no time to try to convince your physician or other staff at the hospital to change their usual procedures. It is simply unrealistic to think you can concentrate on labor and engage in debate at the same time. If there is disagreement between you and hospital personnel, chances are you will lose. Attendants will use measures usual and common for that hospital, including labor, use of drugs, and even cesarean deliveries. Your stated preference will give way to accepted standards of the medical community. Unfortunately, these accepted standards are frequently ill advised and sometimes harmful.

Controlling the use of drugs in labor and delivery. Every obstetrical medication and instrument has possible risks or side effects. Drugs taken by the mother during pregnancy and labor cross the placenta to the baby in varying degrees and amounts. Most drugs used in obstetrics are documented teratogens (Chapter 1). Medications can cause additional complications when the baby is already suffering from prematurity or other abnormalities and can also have undesirable side effects even in a normal, healthy baby. Mothers also suffer various complications and side effects from the use of drugs during labor and delivery. You have the right to know in advance every drug or procedure that will be used during your labor and delivery and should be advised of possible side effects to you and your baby. Accurate records of each medication should be kept during your pregnancy and labor.

Once a woman is in labor, the legal relationship between her and her doctor becomes more complicated. There seems to be a direct relationship between the length of time a woman has been in labor and her loss of control of the situation.[33] This is true partly because of the increase in physical exertion and concentration necessary as labor progresses. The situation is complicated by the horizontal position and by the various tubes and monitoring equipment that severely restrict movement. As contractions intensify, so does powerlessness. Your consent to drugs will be increasingly easy to obtain, as will other interventions your doctor represents as necessary. What your physician will probably not tell you is that most drugs used in obstetrics have not been approved for used in obstetrics and are, therefore, "experimental drugs" in obstetrics. Failure to advice you of this fact may legally negate your consent, leaving grounds for suit. Informed consent for treatment should be obtained before administration of any drug; informed consent for experimentation should be obtained before the administration of any drug not approved for use in labor and delivery.

The FDA approves drugs as safe and effective for a particular use after evaluating potential benefits and risks and determining if the benefits outweigh the risks. The drug may not necessarily be completely safe, but the benefits are considered to outweigh the risks.[34] This assessment does not take into consideration the possible interaction between two or more drugs in the body. This is an extremely complex field of study, and data gathering concerning drug interactions is in its early stages. Recent cases have found physicians and pharmacists liable for failure to warn patients of the possible side effects or for failure to warn them of possible drug interactions.[35]

The few drugs that have been approved for use in labor and delivery, according to their package labels, are alphaprodine (Nisentil), bupivacaine (Marcaine), lidocaine (Xylocaine), meperidine (Demerol), methoxyflurane (Penthrane), and promethazine (Phenergan).[36] Of these, all but bupivacaine were approved between 1938 and 1962, when the standards used by the FDA were of questionable validity. In the summer of 1983, the FDA issued a warning to doctors and hospitals nationwide against giving bupivacaine to women in labor because the drug was suspected of causing 20 pregnant women to die from cardiac arrest. According to the FDA, the cardiac arrests seem to have occurred when the anesthetic was unintentionally injected into a vein rather than just under the skin, a common risk in such injections.

Obstetrical drugs approved before 1962 are now subject to a review for effectiveness by the National Academy of Sciences–National Research Council. This review is limited to effectiveness, however, and does not include safety, which is taken for granted in the absence of reports indicating that the drug is not safe.[36] Even though the FDA requires drug manufacturers to include in the package insert known warnings, contraindications, precautions, and adverse reactions, this requirement does not extend to the physician, as that would interfere, it is claimed, with the practice of medicine. Once the manufacturer has fulfilled requirements of disclosure to the physician, the responsibility and liability for drug-related injuries rests directly with the prescribing physician.

Perhaps the greatest flaw in drug regulation is that a drug may be approved for one purpose and then used for another, rendering the FDA approval virtually meaningless. For example, in 1960, the drug Depo-Provera was approved by the FDA for treatment of endometriosis and terminal endometrial cancer. In 1967, Upjohn submitted an application for use of the drug as a contraceptive injection. Some studies showed a high incidence of mammary tumors in dogs when the drug was administered, and it has never been approved for use as a contraceptive. Nevertheless, many physicians admininstered the drug even though it had not been approved for use as a contraceptive, just as many physicians use drugs in labor and delivery that have not been approved for obstetrical use. Thousands of women were given Depo-Provera, mostly at family planning clinics for people of low income. Its use has now been linked to breast and uterine cancer, sterility, depression, amenorrhea, irregular vaginal bleeding, and fetal defects.[37] The controversy surrounding Depo-Provera is not over. Public hearings were held in the summer of 1983 concerning the FDA's decision not to approve the drug as an injectable contraceptive.[38]

Just as a physician can prescribe an FDA-approved drug for any purpose, a pharmacist may dispense a drug for any purpose. A pharmacist may be legally liable along with the prescribing physician for filling a prescription for a dosage exceeding the package insert recommendations since it is his or her responsibility to see that a prescription conforms to the standards established by the manufacturer for use and dosage.[39]

Current law requires that all drugs with a recognized use in labor and delivery be labeled with available information (or note that the information is not available). The label should show the effects of the drug on the length of labor, increased possibility of forceps or other intervention, increased possibility that resuscitation of the newborn may be necessary, and the effect of the drug on growth, development, and functional maturation of the child. The label must also give information on excretion in the mother's milk and resulting effects on the nursing infant.[37] This information goes only to the doctor. There is no legal requirement that patients must be given the same information. However, patients have the right to have this information before giving their consent to take any medication, and the failure of their physicians to fully inform them of the risks, after being asked, may leave patients with grounds to sue for lack of informed consent. Even over-the-counter drugs must now bear a warning about use by pregnant and nursing mothers.[40]

The FDA for several years proposed to provide patients with information on prescription drugs through the use of patient package inserts. There is no prohibition against patients having access to a drug company's package inserts, and the FDA provides copies to anyone who requests them. Under the proposed regulations, drugs for labor and delivery would have been subject to labeling requirements even though they were administered in a hospital because obstetrical drugs administered as anesthetics are considered "elective." They may be refused by the patient without substantial risks to either mother or unborn child.[41] Because patient labeling information was strongly opposed by many physicians, pharmacists, and drug manufacturers, the proposed regulation was withdrawn.

An Obstetric Care Information Act was recently introduced in the U.S. House of Representatives. This bill would require the states to provide women access to their obstetrical records and would also require the dissemination of current information on obstetrical procedures, specifically the effects and risks of drugs and devices on the health of pregnant women and their developing children. It also provides for a study on the delayed long-term effects on children of obstetrical drugs used by pregnant women. The sponsor of the bill advocates its passage because obstetrical drugs and procedures have never been properly evaluated, and the diethylstilbestrol (DES) experience (p. 96) has served as a drastic example of the need for reform.[42]

The misuse of drugs may be actionable under several legal theories: lack of informed consent, battery, breach of contract, and products liability (to be discussed in the next section). Patients frequently bring suits against hospitals and physicians for injuries caused by the administration of the wrong drug, the wrong dosage, or drugs administered by the wrong route. The injury may be temporary or permanent. Private practitioners are liable for their own negligence in administering a drug and vicariously liable for the negligence of one of their employees. A doctor in partnership is liable for injuries resulting from the negligent administration of a drug by any partner acting within the scope of the partnership. A hospital is liable for the negligence of its employees and may be liable for the negligence of persons not employed by the hospital but using its facilities.[75] As previously mentioned, there are also instances when a pharmacist may be liable for misuse of drugs.

It is of little solace to know that one can sue a drug company for manufacturing a drug that causes cancer or that you can sue your physician for inappropriately prescribing a drug. Women must insist on and seek out all available information about the drugs their doctors prescribe during pregnancy, labor, and delivery. Presently, you have no guarantee that the interests of you and your child are being adequately protected. Past experience illustrates that you cannot rely on your physician, the FDA, or manufacturers to protect you against possibly disastrous effects of obstetrical drugs and procedures.

To protect yourself and your baby and to have the necessary information in case of a later suit, keep an accurate and complete record of all medications prescribed and taken during your pregnancy, including dosage and reason for the prescription. Keep a log during labor (or have your support person do it) that itemizes medication, dosage, and time administered. Otherwise, you will have inadequate information about the drugs to which you and your baby were exposed. Hospitals are generally required to keep complete medical records for patients. Although hospital records are the property of the hospital, a patient has the right to certain information contained in those records. The amount of information depends on the state in which the patient is hospitalized. In all states, the patient has a right to review information relating to admission, history, diagnosis, and discharge. In some states, patients may be given even more information.[43]

Obstetrical Malpractice

The most likely legal transactions involving pregnancy and childbirth are suits brought because of injury to the mother or child. Often several *legal theories* are used in a given case. Persons who may bring suit include mothers, fathers, infants, guardians of infants, the estates of mothers or infants who have died, and various combinations of these. Most jurisdictions do not recognize a *cause of action* for a child if it is not born alive,[8,44] though this is an emerging cause of action and your state may allow it.[7,45] Parties who may be named as defendants include doctors, nurses, anesthesiologists, manufacturers, retailers, clinics, hospitals, midwives, childbirth educators, and genetic counselors.

Most malpractice suits involve multiple plaintiffs and defendants. For example, the mother and child may bring suit against the hospital and several doctors. Occcasionally, a suit is brought by many persons who have joined in a *class action* with common issues and defendants. Recently, federal courts have allowed class action suits by DES victims against drug manufacturers. This kind of consolidation allows plaintiffs to combine resources so that they can afford, as a single plaintiff could not, expert legal assistance and the use of expensive medical experts to develop a case. Class actions help reduce the power differential between the medical consumer and the large insurance companies who often defend such suits.

All states limit the time within which a malpractice suit may be brought through *statutes of limitations*. This limit is often 2 years but varies depending on the state and the legal theory used. Some suits are based on several theories, and recovery may be allowed under some theories and not others. In some states the statute of limitation is extended by the use of a *discovery rule*, meaning that the period during which you may bring suit does not begin until the discovery of the injury. Many states *toll the period* during a person's minority so that suit can be brought after a plaintiff reaches adult years. Courts may also toll the period if the patient fails to discover the cause of the injury as a result of the physician's deception or failure to inform the patient of the true cause of the injury.[46]

Recoverable damages vary depending on the injury, the legal theories used, and state laws governing *malpractice* litigation. Some states limit the total amount of recovery or liability of the defendant, regardless of the degree of negligence or extent of injury. This section discusses the various causes of action that have been successfully used in malpractice obstetrics. Cases of this nature are often settled out of court after prolonged negotiation. Malpractice litigation tends to be very expensive and complicated. Nevertheless, it is increasing, especially in obstetrics.

Assault and Battery; Trespass

Early malpractice litigation was based on assault and battery (unlawful touching) or trespass (an unlawful act causing injury to the person, property, or rights of another). These actions were brought when physician error was rather obvious, such as when the wrong leg was operated on[47] or the physician went beyond the scope of consent during the operation.[48] Recently, a plaintiff brought suit based on the assault theory, claiming the physician failed to warn her of the dangers of oral contraceptives.[49]

Many obstetrical patients complain about behavior by physicians that might be actionable under theories of assault and battery. The following excerpts from letters represent common complaints potentially actionable under the theory of assault and battery:

> When I was approximately 6 weeks pregnant with my daughter, I was involved in a car accident. . . . I was taken to the hospital and given several drugs, among them Thorazine and Valium. I protested that I was pregnant; I was given the drugs regardless and was not given either a pregnancy test or an examination. My daughter was born over 3 weeks late with no apparent problems except for left tibial torsion, which is being treated through the use of a D-B bar and straight last shoes. We cannot stop worrying, however, whether some latent neurological or cardiac problem may occur, since the *Physician's Desk Reference* implies these problems can occur.

• • •

> I was given 50 mg of Demerol and 50 mg of Phenergan when I was just 2 cm dilated, against the expressed wishes of both myself and my husband. . . . Before the doctor arrived, against my protests, she clamped a Penthrane mask on my face.

• • •

> My hands were tied down during delivery.

• • •

> After we finally agreed to the induction, you were very irritated and kept ordering the nurse to turn up the rate of the IV drip, in spite of the fact

that I kept telling you it was too intense. At one point you were in such a snit that you told three separate nurses in a space of 10 minutes to turn the drip up 10 points. Fortunately the nurses had more sense than you and ignored some of your orders. I doubt you meant to turn it up 30 points at a crack, but had they followed your instructions, we'd probably be seeing each other in court. (From a letter to an obstetrician.)

• • •

Contract

A doctor and patient have the same liability to make a contract as do others, and a breach of that contract will give rise to a cause of action. This is separate from a claim in malpractice, though it may arise from the same behavior.[50] In the contract, the physician has expressly agreed either orally or in writing to do a specific thing or occasionally to produce a specific result. A cause of action arises when there has been a breach in the agreement.

Damages that are recoverable under breach of contract are usually limited to payments made and expenditures that flow from the breach, such as costs associated with the operation and treatment, loss of employment, required nursing care, and remedial operations.[50,51] The court in one case found that the plaintiff was entitled to recover for pain and suffering and loss of wages directly resulting from the physician's failure to perform a cesarean section as contracted. In a breach of contract suit, damages might include mental distress and anguish if the contract is personal rather than commercial and if the contract itself is bound up with matters of mental concern.[52]

Breach of contract theory is commonly used in actions against doctors for unsuccessful sterilization procedures. Most courts have allowed such suits even when the plaintiff had a healthy child.[53] (See p. 106 for additional discussion of this cause of action.)

Products Liability

Products liability arises from injury or damages resulting from the use of a product.[54] Suits brought because of injuries caused by health, medical, or hospital supplies may be based on negligence or *strict liability*. Strict liability imposes liability against the seller of the product without regard to a standard of care when a defective product is unreasonably dangerous to the user or consumer. If manufacturers or distributors of health, medical, or hospital supplies do not use reasonable care in the manufacture and marketing of their products and properly warn consumers when they have knowledge of a dangerous or defective condition in the product, an action in negligence exists.[55]

When a mass-produced article or drug is defective, many people can be affected. This is the kind of situation that may be *litigated* as a class action. Several large class action suits are pending that relate to reproduction and childbirth and that have potential impact on millions of women. For example, in 1968 an intrauterine contraceptive device was introduced in the United States. Since then, it has been prescribed to over 2.2 million women. Suits have been filed against the manufacturers, claiming that they were negligent in the design, testing, manufacture, inspection, and distribution of the devices. Alleged injuries include perforation of the uterus, infections of the reproductive organs, pregnancy, spontaneous abortion, fetal injuries, cancer of the uterus, maternal blindness, and loss of consortium. In 1975, 57 separate actions pending in 23 different jurisdictions were consolidated. Defendants in the case include the manufacturer, its personnel, local physicians, clinics, and hospitals.[56]

Suits are often based on strict liability when harmful results have occurred as a result of inappropriate drug prescriptions. In one case, a father brought suit against a pharamaceutical company, claiming that his children were mongoloid as a result of birth control pills prescribed for the mother.[57]

A widely publicized products liability suit involves diethylstilbestrol (DES). DES is a synthetic estrogen that was given to several million women between 1945 and 1971 for the treatment of various complications during pregnancy, most often to prevent miscarriage. Since 1971, the drug has been found to be both teratogenic and carcinogenic. It has been alleged in many suits involving DES that millions of pregnant women were given the drug without being informed that it was experimental. It has never been approved by the FDA to prevent miscarriage.[58] In *Mink v University of Chicago*,[59] it was alleged that patients receiving prenatal care at the University of Chicago Hospital between 1950 and 1952 were given DES in an experiment without their knowledge. A class action suit involving over 1000 plaintiffs was brought against the University of Chicago and Eli Lilly and Company, one of the DES manufacturers, on theories of battery, products liability, and breach of duty to inform. The court allowed the battery action and stated that the manufacturer has a continuing obligation to warn of risks inherent in its drugs based on both strict liability and negligence.[59]

The California Supreme Court broke new legal ground in another DES case when it allowed women to bring a class action suit against drug companies who manufactured DES even though they could not specifically identify which company produced the drugs they took.[61] The plaintiffs claimed, among other things, that DES causes cancerous vaginal and cervical growths in the daughters of mothers given DES during pregnancy and that the various conditions caused by DES do not manifest themselves until at least 10 years after exposure. The suit also alleges that the manufacturers continued to market and advertise the drug even after they had information that it was unsafe and ineffective and that they violated orders of the FDA by marketing DES on an unlimited rather than experimental basis without warning of its potential dangers or that it was experimental.

Another highly publicized products liability case was brought against the manufacturer of Bendectin, an antinausea drug taken by millions of women during pregnancy. Recent scientific studies have suggested that the drug may cause birth defects in 5 out of every 1000 pregnancies. At least 70 suits have been filed in state and federal courts, and the Association of Trial Lawyers of America is actively investigating another 200 possible cases.[62] The drug's manufacturer withdrew Bendectin from the market in the summer of 1983.

Courts seem willing to construe the law to allow these kinds of suits when possible. One case expanded the plaintiff's rights and eased the impact of the discovery rule, since DES damages are often not discovered until many years after the drug was taken. The end result may be more careful screening of drugs used in pregnancy and childbirth and a requirement for more patient information concerning the possible effects of drugs. It emphasizes the necessity for pregnant women to question their doctors about drugs and to maintain accurate and complete information on all drugs (both prescription and nonprescription) taken during pregnancy and delivery because of the impact they may have on their children and on themselves many years later.

Damages recoverable in malpractice are likely to be more extensive and awards larger than with other legal theories. They can include personal injuries, pain and suffering, loss of consortium, estimated losses in the future, medical and other expenses, and future medical expenses.[63] The law recognizes an interest in family relationships, and when negligence has been proven, the recoverable damages may include elements of a familial nature. Early legal recognition of this concept allowed for recovery for loss of services when a family member was injured.[64] The current trend includes more intangible elements such as companionship and affection. If the mother is injured as a result of negligence in the birthing, there may be a cause of action against the physician, nurse, anesthesiologist, hospital, and any other party to the damage on the part of the husband for loss of consortium. Consortium is a bundle of legal rights that includes services, society, sex, and conjugal affection.[65] Another possibility is a claim by the child or older children for loss of care by the parent.[66] In Wisconsin, the state supreme court held that the parents of an infant permanently blinded and disfigured could bring action against a physician for the loss of the injured child's aid, comfort, society, and companionship.[67]

A general rule on money damages is to compensate for all injuries that are a direct and natural result of a breach of duty.[68] How does one prove, in a malpractice case, then, that the physician's care was a breach of duty that would entitle the injured party to an award of damages?

The standard of care and skill that is generally applied in malpractice cases is that which is ordinarily possessed and applied by other doctors in the same community in the same area of practice.[69] If a physician is a "specialist" in some field, the standard usually used is that of a specialist in good standing who is practicing the same specialty in the same locality under similar circumstances.[69] This is referred to as the "locality rule." A physician in a small midwestern town is not held to the same standard as one practicing in a large hospital in New York City. However, several states have rejected the locality rule, finding that there are national standards in the diagnosis and treatment of commonly occurring diseases[70] and that nationally certified medical professionals can be held to a national standard of care.[71]

Most jurisdictions require *expert testimony* to establish the required standard of care as well as the breach of that standard by the defendant. Medical boards have been established to review physician negligence. However, most doctors are reluctant to testify to the negligence of other doctors. Their refusal to do so has been referred to as a "conspiracy of silence."[72]

Traditionally, a hospital has not been liable for acts of physicians who were not actually employed by the hospital. The modern trend is to hold jointly responsible the medical practitioners and the hospitals that permit them to practice.[73] In some states, courts have found as a matter of law that the hospital cannot be held liable for acts of physicians who are *independent contractors*.[74] But in 1978 in Washington, a claim was allowed against a hospital based on the negligent conduct of an emergency room doctor. The court held that the hospital could be held liable under (1) an agency theory, (2) an ostensible agency theory, or (3) directly liable under traditional negligence principles, even though the physician was an independent contractor.[75] Courts are increasingly inclined to find that a hospital is directly responsible to the patient for providing competent medical care and that the failure to screen the medical staff or supervise physicians in certain instances may subject the hospital to liability in malpractice.[76]

Negligence

Medical malpractice is most commonly based on a negligence theory; that is, the physician does not exercise the degree of care and skill that is ordinarily used by the medical profession under similar conditions and circumstances.[77] Negligence is the breach of any legal duty and may involve failure to adequately warn or inform a patient of risks inherent in drugs or procedures, failure to use techniques in an acceptable manner, failure to correctly diagnose conditions, failure to adequately monitor labor, or failure to use the appropriate treatment. For liability to be imposed, there must be (1) a duty owed by the person charged, (2) a breach of that duty, and (3) an injury that is the proximate result of the breach.[78]

Factual settings for suits in negligence include every aspect of childbirth. A New York jury awarded $540,000 to an infant born with severely deformed legs whose mother was unnecessarily treated with eight different drugs during her first trimester of pregnancy.[79] A case was tried before a medical malpractice panel in New York based on the physician's failure to perform a cesarean section that would have been necessary to avoid the infant's oxygen deprivation. As a result, the infant sustained brain damage, among other injuries. The panel held the physician to be negligent, and an $800,000 settlement resulted.[80] Negligence was also asserted in a California case in which there was a delay in the diagnosis and treatment of a prolapsed cord causing anoxia and brain damage. A $17 million settlement was reached.[81]

Numerous suits have been based on the negligent induction of labor. In *Formoff v Means*,[82] a physician persuaded the 20-year-old plaintiff to be induced because of his plans to go out of town. She suffered serious internal injuries relating to the induction, requiring eight major corrective surgeries, including a colostomy and a hysterectomy. A jury awarded $830,000 in damages, including $80,000 to the plaintiff's former husband for loss of consortium. There was a $300,000 settlement for a severely brain-damaged 11-year-old boy whose mother was given Pitocin, which was contraindicated because the baby was presenting in an abnormal (shoulder-arm) position rather than the normal (head first) position.[83]

The negligent use of forceps is another common ground for suit. For example, in Florida, a court held that a claim for malpractice was established by a physician's testimony that the use of Tucker-McLane forceps during a mid forceps delivery constituted a departure from acceptable medical standards.[84] But in New York, a court considering negligence in a forceps case found that when alternative procedures are available and medically acceptable, physicians cannot be held liable in malpractice when they use one of two acceptable techniques.[85]

Frequently, injury in obstetrical malpractice includes emotional trauma or mental distress. Most states require physical injury before damages for emotional trauma can be awarded. California[86] and New York[87] are among a minority of jurisdictions that do not. Although Kentucky law requires that one cannot recover damages for mental anguish unless there is also physical injury, the Kentucky Supreme Court has held that an internist who negligently failed to test for pregnancy before subjecting a patient to x-ray films was liable for her mental and physical pain and suffering when she elected to have an abortion based on a reasonable fear of fetal damage resulting from the radiation.[88]

Damages for mental and emotional distress are being allowed in an increasing number of contexts. For example, damages have been allowed for the psychic injury to a mother resulting from an actual or anticipated tragic birth following negligent conduct.[89] In *Friel v Vineland Obstetrical and Gynecological Professional Association*,[90] a child was negligently and prematurely delivered, causing injury to the mother and child. Even though the child apparently recovered from her injuries, the mother was allowed to sue for damages for anxiety and shock as well as uncertainty about the child's normality during her formative years and until the time when psychological and educational assessment could be conducted.

Abandonment

When a mother alleges complete lack of attendance by her physician during labor, a cause of action exists without a need to present expert testimony. In *Friel*,[90] the woman had suffered serious bleeding before her due date and was told to take aspirin and whiskey. She was finally admitted to the hospital after she became violently ill, suffered convulsions, and continued to bleed. After admission, she was given Demerol and intravenous Pitocin. No one checked on her regularly in the delivery room, and no member of her doctor's group was present at the time of delivery. A physician and hospital were held to be negligent when the physician abandoned the mother and child within 15 minutes after childbirth. The court held that the physician's abandonment was the proximate cause of the infant's resulting brain damage and nervous system damage.[91]

Abandonment by the obstetrician is not uncommon during hospital delivery, as illustrated in these accounts written by mothers.

> For the last 45 minutes, the contractions had no break between them, as they should. The nurse couldn't find you, so she finally turned off the drip herself without permission. (From a letter to the obstetrician.)

• • •

> Later, during the supper hour, I was left alone with one R.N. (my husband was also at supper, nothing, not even ice chips, were permitted by this nurse during labor for either parent), I suddenly knew that the baby was very close. The R.N. just patted my hand and said "keep calm." After another contraction, I told her the baby was coming and she finally decided to listen. Then she left me alone with the stretcher against the bed and an IV bottle in my hand; telling me to get on the stretcher, she went to call the doctor and some help. (From a letter to the authors.)

• • •

> My doctor examined me, burst my water bag. He told my friend I'd be in labor several hours and went out to dinner. Forty-five minutes later I could feel the baby had moved into the birth canal. When the baby crowned, I was moved to delivery and received a "spinal block." Still no doctor. The nurse told me to cross my legs. Agony. Needles in my back. Then another spinal. Finally, doc arrived. Scrub, needle, episiotomy. No one said "push." I assume forceps got him out. Stitch up with eight interns watching over his shoulder. More agony. I was 18, my first child. I wanted to die. It was the worst experience of my whole life. (From a letter to the authors.)

Another mother wrote of her doctor's abandoning her following delivery:

> My doctor never dared to visit me in the hospital for any post-partum checks. I guess he knew how angry I was. (From a letter to the authors.)

Related areas of negligence are failure to obtain an adequate medical history of the mother and failure to communicate information from one attendant to another. In a Kansas case, a jury awarded recovery to a mother who had asked a nurse to call the physician during her labor. The mother was dilated 7 cm and explained to the nurse that she had previously had a very quick birth after 7 cm dilation. The nurse ignored the information, basing her decision not to call the doctor on her own past experiences of labor progress. The physician was not called, the nurse delivered the baby was who in fact born very suddenly, and the mother suffered extensive laceration of the perineum.[92]

Cesarean Deliveries

Between 1968 and 1977, the use of major surgery to deliver babies increased 300% in the United States.[93] Suits involving cesarean births fall into three categories: negligent performance of a cesarean section, failure to perform a timely cesarean section, and performance of an unnecessary cesarean section.[93] Most of these suits arise because of a physician's failure to perform a cesarean delivery in time to avoid preventable injuries. Suits for unnecessary cesarean births are difficult because the plaintiff must be able to show not only that the care provided by the doctor was below acceptable standards but also that the injury was caused by doing the surgical delivery. An error in judgment is not sufficient grounds for suit unless the plaintiff can prove that the course followed by the physician was not an acceptable course followed by a significant segment of the medical community. Cesarean operations are so routinely performed that it might be difficult to prove the last requirement. The proliferation of obstetrical malpractice suits has undoubtedly contributed to the extensive use of cesarean deliveries in the United States.

One court has noted that there is a much higher risk of death to the mother when delivery is surgical rather than vaginal.[94] There is greater risk of maternal mortality caused primarily by anesthetic accidents, hemorrhage, and blood clots.[95] Other cases have held that when a person suffers from a condition from which she will ultimately recover without treatment, proceeding with a treatment that has potential serious risks and where a harmful result occurs is actionable.[96] In this situation, it is not necessary to prove negligence in the procedure itself, only that the risks were significant and the person was unnecessarily exposed to the risks because she would have recovered without the procedure.[97]

There is likely to be an increase in litigation in the area of unnecessary cesarean deliveries because of new information concerning the harmful effects on mother and child of drugs used during surgical delivery, negative psychological effects on the mother when a child is removed surgically, interference in bonding and breastfeeding, and added complications for both mother and child during a cesarean delivery. Possible damages include physical and financial damage resulting from pain and treatment associated with major surgery; costs associated with extensive recuperation such as lost income, child care, and housekeeping assistance; and various forms of mental distress caused by the interruption of bonding and breastfeeding.

Wrongful Birth and Wrongful Life

Some states allow suits for wrongful birth when a doctor's negligence results in a woman's giving birth to a child who would otherwise not have been born. Specifically, the doctor has been sued for negligently performing sterilization or abortion procedures, for failing to inform parents of significant and known genetic risk so they can make the decision to abort, and for failing to diagnose rubella (or other disease) which might lead to a birth defect, in time for the parents to consider a legal abortion.

Courts and juries vary widely on damages allowed in such suits. Parents have recovered for the expense of the unsuccessful operation, attendant pain and suffering, medical complications resulting from the pregnancy, costs of delivery, lost wages, loss of consortium, and mental suffering. Some courts have allowed damages for the estimated cost of raising the child to majority. In Michigan, for example, an appeals court allowed a suit against a physician for negligently misfilling a prescription for birth control pills with a mild tranquilizer, resulting in the birth of a healthy child. The court determined that each of four claimed elements of damage were reasonably ascertainable and the plaintiffs should be allowed to present proof: the mother's lost wages, the pain and anxiety attributable to the pregnancy, the medical and hospital expenses, and the costs of rearing the couple's eighth child.[98]

A Pennsylvania court allowed damages for past and future expenses connected with the birth of a crippled child following a negligent (ineffective) vasectomy but did not allow for the mental and physical suffering of the parents.[99] A New Jersey court came to the opposite conclusion in a similar case. A child was born with *Down's syndrome* to parents who had not been informed of amniocentesis. Damages were allowed for the parents' continuing mental and emotional anguish but not for the costs of rearing the child.[100] An earlier New Jersey decision held that no damages resulted from a failure to inform parents of a possible birth defect so they could consider a legal abortion. The court refused to quantify the difference between life with defects and nonexistence.[101]

"Wrongful life" is an emerging legal doctrine still not recognized by a majority of jurisdictions. It has come about because of the increased effectiveness of diagnostic technology in the area of genetics. Suits in this area have led to the increased use of diagnostic tools such as amniocentesis. Since its use is now common for women over 35 years of age, a physician's failure to inform and/or recommend the procedure to a patient may lead to liability if a child is subsequently born with Down's syndrome or other defects that can be detected through amniocentesis. This is perhaps an unfortunate result because of possible complications with amniocentesis itself, particularly when compared with the statistical possibilities of having a child with Down's syndrome. Again, the key in making a responsible decision concerning the use of amniocentesis is full information comparing the risks of the defects with the risks of the procedure itself and the statistical certainty of the results.

Informed Consent

One of the most controversial theories of medical malpractice involves the failure of physicians to obtain informed consent before proceeding with treatment.[102] The doctrine of informed consent is based on two concepts: the *fiduciary* nature of the relationship between a physician and a patient and the right of a competent person to decide what is to be done to his or her body. In most states, lawsuits concerning lack of informed consent are based on negligence, contending that the doctor is negligent in failing to inform the patient of a known and material risk. Some doctors believe that patients are too ignorant to make decisions on their own behalf and that information increases patients' fears, reinforces "foolish" decisions, and interferes with the faith that patients have in their doctors. Lawyers often take an opposite position, asserting that patients have the absolute right to full and complete information concerning their bodies and what is to be done with them. Many doctors believe that requiring informed consent unduly interferes with professional decision making. Many lawyers believe patients should be making the decisions.[103]

Informed consent has various sources of definition, including constitutional law; federal and state statutes; and individual cases in which courts have defined the term relating to the facts of the case. Generally speaking, informed consent has three elements: capacity, information, and voluntariness.

"Capacity" is the ability to acquire, retain, and use information. Capacity may be affected by age, mental competence, and the situation. A women who is highly drugged or unconscious does not have the capacity to give informed consent.[33]

"Information" should generally include all that a patient needs to know to make a reasoned decision about undergoing a particular procedure. This information includes whether the procedure is diagnostic or therapeutic; whether it requires an incision; duration; need for anesthetic; instruments to be used; how the procedure is to be performed; anticipated outcome; benefits (for example, whether full or only partial relief is anticipated); alternatives, including no treatment; and the risks involved in all alternatives.[104] *How* the information is communicated is probably as important as *what* is communicated. Because of the physician's powerful position, the way in which he or she presents the information, including emphasis, demeanor, and choice of terms, strongly influences a patient's decision. The physician often discloses the information in such a way as to ensure that the patient agrees to treatment.[105] This is particularly meaningful in the obstetrical/gynecological context where 90% or more of the doctors are male and 100% of the patients are women.[106] To quote George Annas, an expert on patient rights, "It is impossible to write an apolitical chapter about the legal rights of women in hospitals. Women are, in fact, at greater risk in hospitals because of the prevailing attitudes of the medical community."[107] Studies have shown that women patients are regarded, and therefore treated, differently than men.[108] Doctors tend to treat women paternally, are more likely to attribute nervous and psychosomatic labels to female complaints, and are less likely to provide full information to women.

"Voluntariness" is an element of consent that also has particular meaning in the obstetrical/gynecological area. To give meaningful consent, a person must be "so situated as to be able to exercise free power of choice without the intervention of any element of force, fraud, deceit, duress, overreaching or other ulterior form of constraint or coercion."[104] This is an interesting problem because once a woman is involved in labor, she is in no position to assert rights or desires not previously made known to the doctor or hospital staff. She is often literally "tied down." If she is denied the company and assistance of a husband or significant other in the labor and delivery room, she is powerless.

The following excerpt from a letter written by an angry mother to her obstetrician concerns informed consent. After the doctor ordered she be given Pitocin to induce labor, the husband questioned the necessity for induction.

> You snapped at him and said that you would not stand for having your medical judgment questioned and that you were in charge and that if he didn't like it we could leave. . . . Saying that we could leave was a really cheap trick. On a cold day it is not practical for a woman with ruptured membranes, partially dilated, to put on wet clothes and go out looking for a new obstetrician. That is not only a cheap thing to do, but it smacks of coercion.

In many cases, the physician fails entirely to inform, much less obtain consent. By way of illustration, one angry mother writes, "My doctor was right in the room and didn't even tell me sugar water was being changed to Pitocin, or why, or was it okay. How dare people give me drugs without my knowledge and consent!"[109]

The doctrine of informed consent has led to numerous malpractice suits when the patient has claimed that consent would not have been given with fuller information. The major areas of dispute are: (1) the scope of the physician's duty to warn, that is, whether the duty is measured by what is normally disclosed by a professional or a general reasonableness standard; (2) whether expert testimony is required to prove the standard of care; and (3) the appropriate test for proving a causal connection between the failure to disclose and the resulting injury. Generally, informed consent is violated if the patient is injured and a jury determines that a *reasonable person* (not the plaintiff, specifically) would have refused treatment if properly informed.[110] Even if a patient can establish a lack of informed consent, he or she must also prove that the failure to inform was the proximate cause of the injury. In other words, the patient must show that had he or she had adequate information, consent to treatment would not have been given and therefore the injury would not have been sustained.

There are four commonly recognized exceptions to the doctrine of informed consent: emergencies, patient incompetence, *waiver* (the patient does not want to participate in the decision), and *therapeutic privilege* (the physician believes that full disclosure would harm or upset the patient). When the risk is the same among several medically acceptable alternatives, the physician has been found to have no duty to compare alternatives for the patient.[111]

At least one court has dismissed an action when the plaintiffs complained that the doctor should have obtained the mother's consent before using low forceps. The child suffered damage to the skull from the forceps delivery. The court pointed out that the use of low forceps in delivery is not hazardous when used with reasonable care, that forceps are routinely used in delivery of babies, and that reasonable medical practitioners do not warn of the risks of low forceps or obtain specific consent for their use.[112] A Florida mother brought a similar suit. The child was delivered by forceps and suffered bruises and lacerations to its head resulting in subdural hematomas. The plaintiff argued that she had not consented to the forceps delivery, the doctor was negligent in using forceps rather than performing a cesarean operation, and the doctor negligently performed the forceps delivery with the wrong type of forceps. In this case, the Florida Supreme Court reversed a lower court's dismissal of the suit, allowing the plaintiff to present evidence as to the defendant's negligence.[113]

In *Hall v United States*,[114] a woman suffered severe injuries from a spinal anesthetic given during the delivery of her child. The court held that there is no duty to warn a patient of the possible consequences of an anesthetic since all anesthetic drugs are inherently dangerous to some degree. All experts testified that most patients are in a state of high anxiety before such a procedure, and it would be bad practice to voluntarily warn a patient of potential adverse effects. (This is an example of the therapeutic exception to informed consent.) The experts also agreed that a doctor should discuss the matter in detail *if asked* by the patient. In other words, the doctors seemed to feel an obligation to answer questions when asked, but no obligation to volunteer information. The clear import of the case is to ask questions about everything.

Signing a consent form is not conclusive in terms of a court's determination that informed consent was made. In Maryland, a woman signed, without reading, a standard hospital consent form 10 to 15 minutes before being wheeled into the delivery room. Her illiterate husband signed the same form. The court held that the signed consent form was not conclusive but merely evidence that could be presented to a jury on the question of consent.[115]

In spite of the concern doctors have expressed over the impact that the informed consent doctrine might have on malpractice litigation, a nationwide survery conducted by the National Association of Insurance Companies showed that failure to obtain informed consent was the basis of only 3% of malpractice claims.[116] The Patient's Bill of Rights (see Appendix G) specifically states that the patient has the right to receive from the physician all information necessary to give informed consent before the start of any treatment. Insisting on and seeking out information is probably the single most important means of avoiding damage to yourself and your child.

In 1982 a survey of 1250 patients and 800 physicians was conducted by Louis Harris and Associates concerning informed consent forms. It showed that 79% of the patients and 55% of the physicians believed that the primary purpose of the form is to protect physicians against lawsuits. Another interesting finding was that 96% of patients said they wanted to know everything, but only 17% of physicians believed that all their patients wanted to know everything.[117]

Right to Refuse Treatment

The right to refuse treatment is a facet of the informed consent doctrine that needs further discussion. It is usually considered in the context of the terminally ill patient's right to refuse extraordinary life-prolonging measures. Nevertheless, it is probably as important in other health care areas and especially in obstetrics. After all, labor and delivery of a child are normal functions that tend to be successfully completed in the great majority of cases without the necessity of intervention. A laboring mother should have the option of proceeding with "normal labor" without routine intervention.

Recent court decisions have held that both the common law and the Constitution protect an individual's right to refuse medical treatment.[118] A model act has been proposed to standardize and implement this important right and could be construed to include obstetrical care.[119] The language of the act refers to actions taken to diagnose, assess, or treat a "disease, illness, or injury," which would seem to exclude childbirth. However, as has been previously noted, at least one court has found that assisting in childbirth is the practice of medicine, thereby presumably finding pregnancy a "sickness or affliction" as defined by California statute.[6]

The right to refuse treatment necessarily has an adjunct—the acceptance of responsibility by the patient for the results of that refusal.

According to the terms of the model act, a physician who declines to follow the patient's wishes must transfer the patient to a physician who will. Health care providers who follow the guidelines would be relieved of legal liability. Those who abandon their patients or refuse to comply would be subject to sanctions, including civil suits in negligence and battery and/or administrative actions such as license suspension or revocation and disciplinary action by licensing boards.

Increasing scientific information is available to show that many of the procedures and interventions commonly and routinely used in labor and delivery are unnecessary and sometimes dangerous. This situation is not confined to obstetrics and gynecology. In 1973, a major study of health care was conducted by the Department of Health, Education and Welfare.[120] One of its findings was that a substantial percentage of adverse medical outcomes occurs *because* of treatment. Surgical and drug intervention and even hospitalization itself carry with them complication rates that must be considered in an overall treatment plan. Several successful suits have been brought against hospitals and staff because of hospital-acquired infections in both mother and child after delivery.[121]

There is evidence that the frequency of iatrogenesis (undesirable side effects of medical intervention) has increased in the past 20 years. Some of the suggested causes include routine monitoring, which, if not accurately assessed, leads to earlier and increased intervention; greater reliability on drugs; and greater use of therapeutic procedures in general. As more technology becomes available, there is a tendency for physicians to use it not only because of a desire to stay current in their field but also because of a legitimate fear of malpractice suits if they do not use the most advanced technology available, even though new technology carries with it new sets of risks and complications.

The concept of right to refuse treatment could play a part in future cases in which a parent has chosen the option of home birth over hospitalization, even though not attended by a legally licensed attendant. Assuming the mother is not in any of the high-risk categories that would preclude a safe home birth, the decision for home birth without the emergency equipment that is available at a hospital should remain the parent's option. Obviously, in light of judicial precedent of considering the unborn child's rights superior to the mother's (as discussed earlier), it may be that the only effective means of refusing treatment is in the home birth setting.

Frivolous Lawsuits

No chapter concerning the legal aspects of childbirth would be complete without a discussion of frivolous lawsuits. Ours is a litigious society, and litigation is one means of bringing about necessary changes. However, the intent of this chapter is not to encourage lawsuits but to inform the reader of possible grounds for suit when appropriate and, it is hoped, to help the reader avoid the necessity of suit. Every error in medical judgment is not legally actionable nor is every bad result the fault of the health care provider.

Legitimate suits are important because a finding in favor of the plaintiff can cushion the financial impact on an individual family for a child who will require a lifetime of specialized care and because it positively affects the future conduct and procedures of medical personnel. Frivolous lawsuits, on the other hand, are extremely costly to our society for several reasons. Because of the proliferation of lawsuits against obstetricians/gynecologists, physicians are forced to pay extremely high premiums for malpractice insurance. This cost is, of course, passed on to the consumer and contributes significantly toward the overall increase in health care costs.

Numerous lawsuits have been brought against physicians for not performing ultrasound, not using electronic fetal monitoring, and not performing cesarean deliveries, making physicians much more likely to practice "defensive" medicine by using these procedures routinely to protect himself or herself. A physician is more likely to be successfully sued for failure to perform a cesarean section than for performing an unnecessary one. Therefore, in making a medical judgment as to whether and when to perform a cesarean delivery (or use ultrasound, electronic fetal monitoring, and other high-tech devices), most doctors will use the procedure and use it earlier than they would if the fear of malpractice did not enter the picture.

Diony Young, in her book *Changing Childbirth*, expresses the view that most obstetrical lawsuits are frivolous and are filed primarily because of a poor relationship between patient and physician, a poor result regardless of cause, or excessive costs. Perhaps the most significant factor is the lack of a good relationship between the patient and the doctor. As more options become available to prospective parents in terms of childbearing facilities and attendants, this situation should improve. Parents educated in all aspects of childbirth trends are more likely to be able to experience the birth they desire by making informed decisions and then taking responsibility for the outcome.

Plan Ahead

Suing your obstetrician (or others) can never remedy the damages done to you and your child during pregnancy or childbirth. Prevention is always worth more than an inadequate and impartial cure. Prevention is not always possible, however, as is illustrated by the experience of thousands of women given DES without their knowledge during the 1950s. But all women who are even considering childbirth should educate themselves fully about their mother's gynecological history, their own medical history, current literature on pregnancy and childbirth, alternative settings and attendants available in the community, and statistics that speak to complications and risk factors of pregnancy.

Women are exerting more control over the birth experience. This increased control is manifested in changing policies, however slowly. Certain areas of the country and certain hospitals have responded more quickly to consumer demands. If possible, you should seek out these facilities.

Not only can an informed mother greatly reduce risks to herself and her baby; she also serves as a consumer advocate for all women. The following are some ways of bringing about changes in obstetrical care:

1. By choosing intelligent and safe alternatives to high-tech birth.
2. By questioning doctors and hospital personnel about standard procedures that are commonly used but that are unnecessary or harmful or that impede labor; by being informed about these matters and then insisting on changes.
3. By reading carefully all consent forms and refusing to sign those that seem to give the physician unlimited discretion.
4. By having an advocate (husband or friend) with you to confer with throughout your prenatal care and birthing who will support your preferences, particularly after you are in labor.
5. By keeping complete and accurate records of all medication and treatment received during prenatal care and during labor.
6. By discussing fully with your doctor before labor your preferences with respect to procedures and medications, his or her

preferences of the above, and his or her preferred or usual means of dealing with contingencies such as prolonged labor, breech presentation, or prolapsed cord.

7. By asking to have your written preferences attached to your medical chart for reference during labor.

8. By recognizing that you are ultimately responsible for the outcome of the birth by making informed choices and by realizing that you can control your baby's environment and introduction to life.

9. By preparing for your child's birth before pregnancy through diet and exercise and through learning about the physiological changes that occur during pregnancy.

Perhaps the most important suggestion is to maintain the attitude that you will control the birthing experience. The above suggestions do not guarantee that you will have an ideal birthing, but they will definitely contribute to your chance of having a birth that is meaningful and manageable, both physically and psychologically. If you have made the above preparations and have a bad result through negligence, you will have the understanding and documentation necessary to sue successfully.

7

Changing Maternity Care:
Consumer Power

Consumer power has been one of the most remarkable forces for changing maternity care in the 1970s and 1980s. Parents, advocates, women's groups, and childbirth groups have found numerous ways to put pressure on the health care system, on physicians, on organized medical groups, on legislatures, on health planning agencies, and on hospitals.[1,2] This chapter describes how the process of consumer advocacy and activism has combined with other factors to change maternity care, the new challenges facing us in the 1980s, and strategies that parents and consumer advocates can use to change the system.

In previous chapters we have seen how the maternity care marketplace has expanded, despite massive opposition from many directions representing power, money, and organization. To try to put a stop to the out-of-hospital birth movement, for example, the opposing groups have used every strategy they could—legislation, harassment, restraint of trade, lawsuits, coercion, denial of care, peer pressure, revocation of professional hospital privileges, insurance penalties, legal threats, violations of the Hippocratic oath, and public abuse.

But, despite it all, the face of childbirth has changed. As a result, families today have infinitely more choices available to them than they had 15 years ago. Paralleling those family-centered changes, however, has been the increasing reliance on obstetrical technology, which

---

Portions of this chapter are adapted from Young, D.: Changing childbirth: family birth in the hospital, Rochester, N.Y., 1982, Childbirth Graphics, Ltd., Chapters 23 and 24.

threatens to engulf the event of birth. This does not mean we must reject the advances in obstetrical and newborn technology, but it does mean we must reject their unnecessary use. And we owe it to ourselves and to our children to take up the challenge of finding the ways out of this trap of technology.

Stimulus for Change

Family-centered childbirth was the rare exception in North American hospitals before 1970. However, a fortuitous combination of factors began to gnaw away at traditional maternity care in the early 1970s, thus launching the decade of change in maternity care.[1] What were these factors that precipitated the new trend toward a more humanized and personalized system of maternity care?

First, dissatisfied parents began to apply pressure directly on doctors and hospitals. Parents were becoming much better informed about all aspects of childbirth by attending childbirth education classes. Often they found that their plans for a prepared childbirth were thwarted once they stepped inside the hospital doors. Their cause was taken up by outspoken consumer advocates who began to publicly criticize the maternal health system. The very titles of their books—*The Cultural Warping of Childbirth,*[3] *Forced Labor,*[4] and *Immaculate Deception*[5]—told the childbearing public that all was not well in obstetrical care. Not only did they write books, they addressed meetings, used the media, and raised the consciousness of both parents and professionals. At the same time the women's movement was also beginning to question all areas of women's rights, including how they related to women's health care.[6]

Second, there was a revival of interest in alternative birthing, both in and out of the hospital. New, family-centered birth settings in a few hospitals set the stage for competition for the maternity client. Other families decided to have their babies at home. At the same time, a resurgence of interest in midwives added a welcome new option for parents in choosing a provider of maternity care, as well as putting additional competitive economic pressure on obstetricians. The first freestanding birth center opened in New York City in 1975, beginning an exciting new advance in low-risk, low-technology childbirth that was removed from the acute care hospital. The marketplace was expanding for families.

Third, pioneering research on mother-infant and father-infant bonding showed that parents and newborns benefitted when they were not separated in the immediate newborn period.[7] Newborn behavior studies also provided exciting insights and information about infant responses in the early hours and days after birth.[8] Science was at last proving what parents had instinctively known for years! Here was the evidence that supported family togetherness at birth.

Fourth, national medical, obstetrical, pediatric, and nursing organizations began to respond to the consumer pressure and scientific evidence and to reexamine traditional care practices and philosophies. The concept and practice of family-centered care were endorsed and supported in position papers and professional documents, further stimulating hospitals to introduce change.[9-12]

Thus the stage was set for a revolution in maternity care.

Consumers Speak Out

Parents and childbirth advocates realized that the health care system was there to serve them, and as buyers of maternity care and services, they needed to get involved and take action if their needs and demands were going to be met.[1,2]

Although there were concerned maternal health professionals who saw the need for change and initiated efforts to make the system more sensitive to the family's emotional and social needs, the fire, the energy, and the push had to come from the public. And it did. Individual parents began to read and inform themselves about childbirth and obstetrical practices and technology. They questioned many of the unscientific and unproved procedures and treatment, and a few brave ones changed doctors, hospitals, and even towns and states to have the kind of birth they wanted. Yet others abandoned hospitals altogether.

Not only were individual parents beginning to assert themselves, but others were taking direct steps to bring about changes through a wide variety of strategies. As these advocates and pioneers began to speak out, they found some responsive professional ears. Progressive hospitals started to listen and take a hard look at some of their long-held and often unscientific policies and practices.[1]

National groups that advocated childbirth options, alternative birth settings, family-centered maternity care, and childbirth education launched stronger efforts to humanize maternity care and push for birth alternatives. New organizations sprang up, such as home birth groups, breastfeeding groups, midwifery support groups, parent support groups, cesarean prevention groups, and childbirth choice groups. They devoted their energies to changing specific areas of maternal and newborn health care.

When public hearings were held on obstetrical practices, midwifery, consolidation of maternity services, and maternal and child health care, consumer advocates, parents, and groups appeared to testify. They pressed their legislators to hold hearings on particularly controversial issues.

Childbirth conferences and meetings were organized that focussed on birth alternatives, where people could share strategies and plan ways of bringing about change. The massive walls of traditional maternity care were being breeched, and it was essential to inspire others with the spirit to go to work in their communities.

The Clouds Ahead

Maternity care was indeed moving forward, but other, more ominous trends were beginning to surface, presenting new challenges. The 1970s ushered in a whole new technology in obstetrics, and it was being applied to childbearing women with enthusiasm and often without valid reason.[13,14]

The cesarean birth rate more than tripled in a decade, going from 5.5% of all births in 1970 to 17.9% in 1981.[15] Electronic fetal monitoring became routine in many hospitals. Epidural anesthesia increased in popularity, and the 12-hour labor appeared on the horizon, following the practice in Dublin, Ireland, where all primigravidas are required to give birth by the end of 12 hours of labor.[16] Ultrasound use was becoming more common as doctors bought the revolutionary new equipment for their private offices. The routine use of other interventions such as IVs, medications, and episiotomies continued unabated at many hospitals.

Now the specter of malpractice hovers over the entire practice of medicine. The fear of a lawsuit, filed by parents or baby for a poor birth outcome, has persuaded obstetricians to cover themselves by using more and more tests and technology.[17,18] Defensive obstetrics is a reality of the 1980s, pushing up malpractice premiums for doctors, midwives, nurses, and hospitals and increasing health care costs for us all.[18,19]

Unfortunately, in their eagerness to jump on the bandwagon of family-centered maternity care, many hospitals fail to realize that it is more a philosophy and attitude than it is color-coordinated furnishings, carpeting, and hanging plants. Today, many hospitals only pay lip-service to the practice of family-centered care, and the image does not meet the reality. Rigid regulations and restrictive practices are commonplace. Many birthing rooms and centers are vastly underutilized because of staffing problems, resistance from doctors and nurses, and too rigid screening criteria for eligible families.[20]

The 1980s must also face the problem of physician oversupply. There are just too many doctors, especially specialists in the field of obstetrics. Economic competition for the childbearing client is becoming more fierce, and increasingly midwives, family physicians, and female obstetricians are becoming the target of restraint-of-trade efforts.[21] Alternative birth settings, such as home births and freestanding birth centers, provide additional economic threats to the medical system.

Parents, consumer advocates, and childbirth groups must now move on many fronts to deal with these emerging trends of the 1980s. They must be ever vigilant to see that the progressive policies and practices adopted by hospitals do not degenerate into tokenism and illusion. It is a sad fact that the majority of hospitals are more concerned with meeting their own institutional needs than they are with meeting the needs of those they serve. We must therefore continue to apply pressure to make hospitals and health providers accountable to the public.

Change Strategies

The question is: How can each of us make the maternity system better and more responsive to what we want? Why should you bother to make the effort, you might wonder? Simply, because it is your body, your health, your baby, your community, your hospital, and your money. In every way, you have a stake in your maternity system, and at all levels of participation you have a responsibility to do something.

First, this means doing something for yourself, which requires rejecting the role of patient, to which you have been conditioned for so long, and taking on the active role of helping yourself to have a healthy birth outcome and to have the kind of birth you want. You need, therefore, to reject the medical and pathological model of pregnancy and birth and to acknowledge that pregnancy, labor, and birth are healthy, physiological processes and that your body is capable of doing the job of giving birth. You need to gather all the information you can to help you take care of yourself and your fetus and to tune your mind and body for the work ahead.

Find out in advance everything you can about childbirth—where to go, who to see for your care and for childbirth education classes, what to ask, and what your choices are. Shop the marketplace, read, ask questions, and explore the alternatives. Go to childbirth education classes and look around for ones that are consumer oriented and discuss alternatives. Hospital classes will be more provider oriented and supportive of the medical model of childbirth.

Learn about your rights and responsibilities in childbirth and exercise your right to change birth practitioners or facilities if you are not satisfied. Read and find out about obstetrical procedures, treatment, practices, and drugs—when they should be used, what they can do to help, what are their risks, and what you could do instead. With all this information, you and your partner can make a birth plan to describe what you want and don't want and then discuss and negotiate your choices and preferences with your doctor or midwife. If you find that you and your birth practitioner are not in tune with each other (and a birth plan can be threatening to a traditionally minded doctor) or if your hospital does not offer what you want, go elsewhere. However, be sure that you let them know why you are seeking care somewhere else, because eventually the message may get through and they may decide to do something about changing attitudes and practices.

Often, it isn't until after the birth, with the experience fresh in your mind, that you may decide to speak out and take action to persuade a hospital or health system to introduce changes. What are some of the consumer strategies that have proved effective?

Face-to-face meetings with hospital personnel. Such meetings provide the advantage of shared participation and communication, immediate feedback, clarification of issues, and a captive audience. Write a letter and ask to have a meeting with the chiefs of obstetrics and pediatrics, the nursing supervisor, administrator, and public relations director. In your letter, introduce yourself or your group and describe the policy or practice you would like reexamined or suggest they consider establishing a new program. Include relevant documentation[1] in support of your objective. Send copies of your letter to all those with whom you wish to meet. Be persistent in your efforts to have this meeting; more than one letter may be necessary.

When the time comes, arm yourself with your supporters (a few), your documentation, your courage, your enthusiasm, and your facts.

Discuss the benefits of the policy change or new program—to the family and to the hospital—its safety aspects, cost benefits, how it can be implemented, and need for in-service education of staff. Follow up with a thank-you-for-your-interest letter and keep a close eye on progress. Enlist other parents and groups to write letters in support of your suggestion.

Letters to the hospital. A carefully phrased, constructively written letter to the chief of obstetrics or pediatrics, with copies to the hospital administrator, medical director, and nursing supervisor, can sometimes be amazingly effective in getting a change in policy underway. It helps to start off by praising the hospital for a program or its responsiveness to community input before launching into a description of what you would like changed. You might mention that other hospitals in the community offer this birth option and have found it successful. If you cite support for your suggestion from the medical literature, this can help. You could offer to come in to discuss the matter further, if they wish, and say that you look forward to their reply.

Letters to the newspaper. Hospitals don't like negative publicity. If you have made constructive attempts to communicate your concerns to the hospital and have heard nothing in reply or have been rebuffed, a letter to the editor of the local newspaper, naming the hospital and describing your experience and communications with them, may precipitate action. Be sure of your facts and offer constructive suggestions for addressing the problem.

Petitions. Many groups have readily obtained the names of parents on a petition requesting a change in policy. Childbirth education groups have class participants who might be only too ready to sign a petition. An advertisement in the paper or letter to the editor is also a means to enlist supporters in the community. The petition can then be presented to the hospital administrator. Again, offer to discuss the matter further and keep in contact with the administrator to monitor action.

Press conferences and newspaper articles. Contact the press about major or controversial issues. It helps to find out which reporters work on women's issues and health issues. You can prepare a news release, provide supporting documentation, or hold a press conference with supporters to discuss the issue. Even a phone call to a reporter alerting him or her to a hot issue (for example, an unusually high cesarean birth rate in a local hospital; gross underutilization of a hospital birth center; revoking of, or refusal of, hospital privileges for a local midwife; restrictive labor and birth policies) can prompt an investigation and article.

Group power. You can join the effort to get changes in your community by taking part in the actions of a childbirth group, or you can form your own group. Plan to have the focus one of action rather than discussion and draw up your list of objectives and strategies to get things moving. Joining forces with others can provide moral support and strength, and the workload of obtaining information, writing press releases, or organizing public meetings can be spread around.

Liaisons with providers. It is very helpful to find a sympathetic ally in the hospital you are targeting for change. Often you will find the groundwork has been laid, and this person (nurse or doctor) can suggest appropriate strategies; give inside information about internal politics, power, and organization; provide documentation; advise on timing of your approach; and offer encouragement. Once you have found your ally, make sure you keep in touch regularly to keep on top of what is happening. Other health agencies in the community may provide valuable strategy as well, not to mention information about outcome statistics for a hospital maternity unit or other useful documentation. Offer to help concerned providers in their change efforts.

Directories. Several childbirth or consumer groups have looked at the providers and services in their community and then published a directory. Such a directory can serve as a consumer guide to maternity care, describing where childbearing families can go to have their baby and what services and options are offered. Other groups have published a doctor directory, which allows parents to do comparison shopping by reading the responses by local doctors to a questionnaire about their attitudes and practices. The publication and circulation of such directories have had a stimulating effect on precipitating changes among providers of maternity care and of course have provided expectant parents with invaluable information about what is available in their community.

Joint planning. Often when a hospital plans to renovate its maternity unit, establish an alternative birth center, or initiate new family-centered programs, it appoints a planning task force. If you are aware that innovations are being considered, offer your time and expertise as a childbearing parent to serve on this planning board. The advantages of joint planning are many, but it especially engenders a feeling of respect for concerns on both sides of the issue. The hospital staff learn about what parents want and vice versa. Make sure you are not so intimidated by being in the provider camp that you cannot bring yourself to speak out. For this reason it is a good idea to suggest an additional name or two of consumer representatives for mutual support at the meetings.

Boycotts and demonstrations. When your efforts to bring about change have gone nowhere, the power of boycott can be highly effective. There are many reports of parents moving to another town or state to get a particular birth option they wanted and publicizing their action in the newspaper and on television. Indeed, the mere threat of such action can bring about a reversal of policy amazingly quickly. As already mentioned, hospitals dislike negative publicity and any implication that they are not responsive to community wishes. Even more powerful is a demonstration with multitudes of placard-waving parents in front of a hospital. In April, 1982, in London, there was an incredible demonstration of parent power as 5000 people paraded in front of a large hospital to protest restrictive labor and delivery practices. One well-known childbirth educator, Sheila Kitzinger, said that childbirth in Britain will never be the same! The time may come when a demonstration may be the only avenue left to get the hospital to listen and take action.

Political and legislative arenas. Use your legislators and your power as lobbyists to get changes in maternal and child health legislation. Changing an outdated or restrictive health regulation or trying to establish a freestanding birth center could be a valuable objective for a childbirth group. Rally support from other groups or consumer advocates. Initiate new legislation, but you will need to familiarize yourself with the political process in your state or province before you begin.[22] When public hearings are held at state or national levels on issues of maternal and child health, prepare a statement and give testimony, either as an individual or as a representative of a group. Make your government health agencies and legislators aware of your existence by making yourself highly visible and verbal.

Resistance to Change

Be prepared for a variety of resistance tactics and power plays when you become a pioneer for changing maternity care.[23] Not only can the fact that you are an outspoken consumer be highly threatening, but the very idea of change and innovation is a threat to a person's sense of security and to values, beliefs, attitudes, economic status, prestige, power, and traditions.[1] Changing attitudes is one of the first and most difficult tasks facing you, and you will have to call on all your negotiating strategies and skills. Once attitudes have been changed, the chances of action are greatly increased.

Several "tricky tactics" may be used to throw you off balance and divert you from your goal, including the use of deliberate deception, psychological warfare, and positional pressure tactics.[24] Therefore, you must be prepared to deal with these ploys.

Deliberate deception includes misrepresentation of facts or intentions and withholding useful information,[24] such as lines of authority, procedures, dates of meetings, or other in-house actions. For example, one group reported that they were put off with provider control of timing for consumer input.[23] Excuses were given such as, "It's too soon for public participation," "The time's not right," "Let's wait until the staff has had a chance to work on the problem," or "The meeting to discuss that was held last month."

Psychological warfare may include deliberate personal attacks, insulting behavior which implies that you are ignorant and have no valid contribution to offer, holding meetings on provider turf in stressful surroundings, or threats.[23,24] For example, childbirth educators who rock the boat or teach about birth options have received letters threatening refusal to refer expectant parents to their classes.

Positional pressure tactics may include refusal to communicate, negotiate, or meet with you or your group; playing you off against your peers; using delaying tactics; or controlling the rules of the game.[24] For example, a carefully orchestrated game plan may be in place, including preselected topics for discussion, a set agenda, and other barriers to your participation.[23]

Recognize these tactics if they are used, raise them openly and explicitly, and question the legitimacy of using them.[24] In other words, don't let them get away with it—call them on their action. Stick to your issue, keep your cool, and don't attack people personally. Suggest an alternative way of going about the problem for mutual satisfaction.[24]

Plan your action strategies ahead so if one doesn't work you can move on to the next strategy, and the next, until you stand "if necessary, outside the hospital itself, picket in hand!"[1] The road may be long, rocky, and hard, but if you're persistent, you will find a way to get what you want. Persistence is the key to success. Each action you take to challenge and change the maternity system opens the door further and frees childbearing families from the meshes of medicalized childbirth. The time for action is now!

Notes

Chapter 1

1. Wertz, R.W., and Wertz, D.C., Lying-in: a history of childbirth in America, New York, 1977, The Free Press.
2. American College of Obstetricians and Gynecologists, Committee on Maternal Health: National study of maternity care; survey of obstetric practice and associated services in hospitals in the United States, Chicago, 1970, U.S. Maternal and Child Health Services.
3. Haire, D.B., Perinatal maternal mortality rates by size and type of hospital. In Stewart, D., and Stewart, L., eds.: Safe alternatives in childbirth, Marble Hill, Mo., 1976, NAPSAC Reproductions.
4. Hospitals have always had high rates of infection, but the introduction of antibiotics at the end of the 1930s drastically cut the frequency with which infected patients died. Infection rates in hospital obstetrical services have increased, however, during the last decade.
5. Fleck, A., Personal communication.
6. Marieskind, H. I., An evaluation of caesarean section in the United States, final report submitted to U.S. Department of Health, Education and Welfare, 1979, 311-234/4 1-3, Washington, D.C., 1980, U.S. Government Printing Office. Note that there is also wide variation in cesarean section rates for individual physicians. Rates for board certified obstetricians/gynecologists are the highest (25% to 50%) while rates for family practice physicians are much lower (10% to 20%).
7. Ratner, H.: The history of dehumanization of American obstetrical practice. In Stewart, D., and Stewart, L., eds.: 21st century obstetrics now!, vol. 1, Marble Hill, Mo., 1977, NAPSAC Reproductions.
8. Horowitz, S.: Personal communication, Blue Cross & Blue Shield.
9. Riley, E.M.D.: What do women want?—the question of choice in the conduct of labour. In Chard, T., and Richards, M., eds.: Benefits and hazards of the new obstetrics, London, 1973, Heinemann Medical.
10. Kantor, H.I., and others: Value of shaving the pudendal-perineal area in delivery preparation, Obstet. Gynecol. 25:509–512, 1965.
11. Romney, M.L.: Predelivery shaving: an unjustified assault? Obstet. Gynecol. 1:33, 1980.

12. Feldman, S.: Choices in Childbirth, New York, 1978, Grosset & Dunlap.
13. Birnbaum, D.A., The iatrogenesis of damaged mothers and newborns. In Stewart, D., and Stewart, L., eds.: 21st century obstetrics now!, vol. 1, Marble Hill, Mo., 1977, NAPSAC Reproductions.
14. Study finds enema in labor need not be routine, Ob. Gyn. News **16**(14):40, 1981.
15. Romney, M.L., and Gordon, N.: Is your enema really necessary? Br. Med. J. **282**:1269, 1981.
16. Flynn, A.M., and others: Ambulation in labour, Br. Med. J. **26**:591, 1978.
17. Sparrow, L., An open letter to the OB Department at Beth Israel Hospital, Boston, Reprinted with permission from NAPSAC News, **7**(2):17, 1982.
18. Rindfuss, R.R., and Ladinsky, J.L., Patterns of births: implications for the incidence of elective induction, Med. Care **14**:685, 1976. This article presents an interesting sociological analysis of the "weekend birth deficit."
19. Chalmers, I., and Richards, M., Intervention and causal inference in obstetric practice. In Chard, T., and Richards, M., eds.: Benefits and hazards of the new obstetrics, London, 1977, Heinemann Medical. Strangely enough, however, even when the United Kingdom induction rate increased by 50%, the proportion of postmature babies did not decrease.
20. Niswander, K.R., and Gordon, M., The women and their pregnancies, U.S. Department of Health, Education and Welfare, The Collaborative Perinatal Study of the National Institute of Neurological Diseases and Stroke, DHEW Pub. No. (NIH) 73–379, Washington, D.C., 1972, U.S. Government Printing Office.
21. Recently, the FDA officially frowned on using oxytocin for elective induction, that is, induction for convenience. This means that hereafter labor will be electively induced by other substances such as prostaglandins or by amniotomy followed by oxytocin.
22. Howie, P.W., Induction of labour. In Chard, T., and Richards, M., eds.: Benefits and hazards of the new obstetrics, London, 1977, Heinemann Medical.
23. Some mothers' experiences of induced labour, report to National Childbirth Trust, London, 1975. Cited in Corea, G., The hidden malpractice: how American medicine mistreats women, New York, 1977, Jove.
24. Yudkin, P., and others: A retrospective study of induction of labour, Br. J. Obstet. Gynaecol. **83**:257, 1976.
25. Blacow, M., and others: Induction of labour, Lancet **1**:217, 1975.
26. Goldenberg, R.L., and Nelson, K.: Iatrogenic respiratory distress syndrome: an analysis of obstetric events preceding delivery of infants who develop respiratory distress syndrome, Am. J. Obstet. Gynecol. **123**:617, 1975.
27. Caldeyro-Barcia, R.: Some consequences of obstetrical interference, Birth Fam. J. **2**:34, 1975.
28. Oski, F.A.: Oxytocin and neonatal hyperbilirubinemia, Am. J. Dis. Child. **129**:1139, 1975.
29. Fields, H.: Induction of labor: methods, hazards, complications and contraindications, Hosp. Top. **46**:63, 1968.
30. Fields, H.: Induction of labor: its past, its present, and its place, Postgrad. Med. p. 226, 1968.
31. Lumley, J.: Antepartum fetal heart rate tests and induction of labour. In Young, D., ed.: Obstetrical intervention and technology in the 1980s, Women Health **7**:9, 1982.
32. Simkin, P.P.: Amniotomy. In Young, D., ed.: Obstetrical intervention and technology in the 1980s, Women Health **7**:103, 1982.

33. Is fetal monitoring safe?, Washington Post, p. 3, April 16, 1978.
34. Every woman probably should be monitored during labor, *Ob. Gyn. News* **17**(20):1, 1982.
35. Banta, H.D., and Thacker, S.B.: Costs and benefits of electronic fetal monitoring: a review of the literature, U.S. Department of Health, Education and Welfare, National Center for Health Services Research, DHEW Pub. No. (PHS) 79–3245, Washington, D.C., 1979, U.S. Government Printing Office.
36. Haverkamp, A.D., and Orleans, M.: An assessment of electronic fetal monitoring. In Young, D., ed.: Obstetrical intervention and technology in the 1980s, Women Health **7**:115, 1982.
37. Although impatience and nervousness may contribute to hasty decisions to do a cesarean section, the real culprit may be an excessive amount of data stemming from the fact that electronic fetal monitoring goes on continuously rather than periodically, as in manual monitoring. The logic of this argument is as follows: The decision to do a surgical delivery rests on the occurrence of abnormal heart rate patterns. The frequency with which abnormal heart rate patterns are detected is a function of the total volume of heart rate data. Continuous monitoring yields more data than periodic monitoring. Therefore, from a purely statistical point of view, continuous monitoring will result in more cesarean sections than will periodic monitoring.
38. Hellegers, A.E.: Fetal monitoring and neonatal death rates, N. Engl. J. Med. **299**:357, 1978.
39. Banta, H.D., and Thacker, S.B.: Assessing the costs and benefits of electronic fetal monitoring, Ob/Gyn Survey **35**:627, 1979.
40. Ettner, F.M.: Hospital obstetrics: do the benefits outweigh the risks. In Stewart, D., and Stewart, L., eds.: 21st century obstetrics now!, vol. 1, Marble Hill, Mo., 1977, NAPSAC Reproductions.
41. Gassner, C.B., and Ledger, W.J.: The relationship of hospital-acquired maternal infection to invasive intrapartum monitoring techniques, Am. J. Obstet. Gynecol. **126**:33, 1976.
42. Cetrulo, C.L., and Freeman, R.K.: Problems and risks of fetal monitoring. In Aladjem, S., ed.: Risks in the practice of modern obstetrics, St. Louis, 1975, The C.V. Mosby Co.
43. Herpes at electrode site an added risk of fetal monitoring, *Ob. Gyn. News* **16**(20):12, 1981.
44. Supine called the worst position for labor and delivery, Fam. Pract. News **5**:11, 1975.
45. Dunn, P.M.: Obstetric delivery today: for better or for worse, Lancet **1**:792, 1976.
46. Narroll, F., Narroll, R., and Howard, F.H.: Position of women in childbirth: a study in data quality control, Am. J. Obstet. Gynecol. **82**:943, 1961.
47. Corea, G.: The hidden malpractice: how American medicine mistreats women, New York, 1977, Jove.
48. Howard, F.H.: Delivery in the physiologic position, Obstet. Gynecol. **11**:318, 1958.
49. Bienarz, J., and others: Aortocaval compression by the uterus in late human pregnancy: II. An arteriographic study, Am. J. Obstet. Gynecol. **100**:203, 1968.
50. Goodlin, R.C.: Aortocaval compression during cesarean section: a cause of newborn depression, Obstet. Gynecol. **37**:702, 1971.
51. Humphrey, M., and others: The influence of maternal posture at birth on the fetus, J. Obstet. Gynaecol. Br. Commonwealth **80**:1075, 1973.

52. Mauk, M.D., and others: Tonic immobility produces hyperalgesia and antagonizes morphine analgesia, Science **213**:353, 1981.

53. Blankfield, A.: The optimum position for childbirth, Med. J. Aust. **2**:666, 1965.

54. Mehl, L.E.: Research on alternatives in childbirth: what can it tell us about hospital practice? In Stewart, D., and Stewart, L., eds.: 21st century obstetrics now!, vol. 1, Marble Hill, Mo., 1977, NAPSAC Reproductions.

55. Wolk, D.J., Student doctors: learning to lie. In Winning essays of the essay contest for students in the health professions, Philadelphia, 1980, Society for Health and Human Values.

56. Haverkamp, A.D., and others: The evaluation of continuous fetal heart rate monitoring in high-risk pregnancy, Am. J. Obstet. Gynecol. **125**:310, 1976.

57. Hourly vaginal exams can detect arrested dilation, Ob. Gyn. News **16**:8, 1981.

58. Brendsel, C., Peterson, G., and Mehl, L.E.: Episiotomy: facts, fictions, figures, and alternatives. In Stewart, D., and Stewart, L., eds.: Compulsory hospitalization: freedom of choice in childbirth?, vol. 1, Marble Hill, Mo., 1979, NAPSAC Reproductions.

59. Obstetrical statistics of the Netherlands. Cited by Mehl, L.E.: Research on alternatives in childbirth: what can it tell us about hospital practice? In Stewart, D., and Stewart, L., eds.: 21st century obstetrics now!, vol. 1, Marble Hill, Mo., 1979, NAPSAC Reproductions.

60. Episiotomy: a surgical procedure, NAPSAC News **6**(3):13, 1981.

61. Chalmers, I., and others: Obstetric practice and outcome of pregnancy in Cardiff residents, 1965–73, Br. Med. J. **1**:735, 1976.

62. Thacker, S.B., and Banta, H.D.: Benefits and risks of episiotomy. In Young, D., ed.: Obstetrical intervention and technology in the 1980s, Women Health **7**:161, 1982.

63. Shy, K.K., and Eschenbach, D.A.: Fatal perineal cellulitis from an episiotomy site, Obstet. Gynecol. **54**:292, 1979.

64. Kitzinger, S., and Walters, R.: Some women's experiences of episiotomy, London, 1981, National Childbirth Trust.

65. Teasdale, C.: Personal communication.

66. Reprinted with permission from NAPSAC News **6**(2):13, 1981.

67. Dobbing, J., and Sands, J.: Quantitative growth and development of the human brain, Arch. Dis. Child. **48**:757, 1973.

68. Brackbill, Y.: Obstetrical medication study, Science **205**:447, 1979.

69. How long do these obstetrical drug effects last? Are the underlying anatomical and physiological effects permanent? In 1979, the FDA admitted that obstetrical drugs do affect newborns adversely, though it hedged on drawing the same conclusion from research with older babies. Nevertheless, most scientists who have tested babies 10 days of age or older have found the same behavioral effects at later ages, long after the drugs have been metabolized and excreted from the body. At these later ages, the behavioral effects are less easily detected, but that does not necessarily mean the underlying anatomical injury has disappeared. Anatomical and histological research with animals whose mothers were administered obstetrical drugs during pregnancy or birth suggests that the damage is indeed permanent.

70. U.S. Food and Drug Administration: Use of drugs for unapproved indications: your legal responsibility, Washington, D.C., 1972.

71. Gintzler, A.R.: Endorphin-mediated increases in pain threshold during pregnancy, Science **210**:193, 1980.

72. Vellay, P.: Painless labour: a French method. In Howells, J.G., ed.: Modern perspectives in psycho-obstetrics, New York, 1972, Brunner/Mazel, Inc.

73. Stewart, D.: Home: the traditional safe place for birth. In Stewart, D., ed.: The five standards for safe childbearing, Marble Hill, Mo., 1981, NAPSAC Reproductions.

74. National Prescription Audit, ed. 16, Forst Washington, Pa., 1977, IMS Press.

75. Woodward, L., and others: Exposure to drugs with possible adverse effects during pregnancy and childbirth, Birth **9:**165, 1982.

76. Doering, P.L., and Stewart, R.B.: The extent and character of drug consumption during pregnancy, J.A.M.A. **239:**843, 1978.

77. Bradley-trained mothers who deliver in-hospital are an exception to these statistics. The *Bradley method* is probably the strongest of all formal methods in advocating avoidance of drugs, with the consequence that 75% to 80% of Bradley-trained mothers who choose to deliver in-hospital do so without resort to prenatal or perinatal medication. However, since Bradley training precedes less than 0.3% of all births in the United States, even if 100% of Bradley-trained women had drugless births, it would still not alter the statistical fact that virtually all hospital births involve the administration of drugs during labor and delivery.

78. Rosengren, W.R., and DeVault, S.: The sociology of time and space in an obstetrical hospital. In Freidson, E., ed.: The hospital in modern society, New York, 1963, The Free Press.

79. U.S. Congress-Senate Subcommittee on Health and Scientific Research: The implications of the elective induction of labor for the health of mothers and children, Statement prepared for hearings on obstetrical practices in the United States by R.R. Rindfuss, April 17, 1978.

80. Rindfuss, R.R., and others: Convenience and the occurrence of births: induction of labor in the United States and Canada, Int. J. Health Serv. **9**(3):439, 1979.

81. Vacuum extractor termed safe, useful for cesarean delivery, Ob. Gyn. News **15**(22):12, 1980.

82. Kitzinger, S., and Davis, J.A., eds.: The place of birth, Oxford, 1978, Oxford University Press.

83. O'Driscoll, K., and others: Forceps cause most of the serious injuries to heads of first born, Ob.Gyn. News **17:**32, 1982.

84. Chalmers, J.A.: The vacuum extractor in difficult delivery, J. Obstet. Gynaecol. Br. Commonwealth **72:**889, 1965.

85. Plauché, W.C.: Fetal cranial injuries related to delivery with the malmstrom vacuum extractor, Obstet. Gynecol. **53:**750, 1979.

86. After Julius Caesar who, according to myth, was surgically delivered.

87. This is true only for the United States. In other countries, most deliveries following a section are normal, vaginal deliveries.

88. Draft Report of the Task Force on Cesarean Childbirth, U.S. Department of Health and Human Services, Public Health Service, National Institutes of Health, Washington, D.C., 1980.

89. Placek, P.J., Taffel, S., and Moien, M.: Cesarean section delivery rates: United States, 1981, Am. J. Public Health **73:**861, 1983.

90. Are primary cesarean section rates too high?, Ob. Gyn. News **16**(22):38, 1981.

91. One study found an average of 15 different drug products administered during cesarean sections.

92. Wilson, J.T., and others: Drug excretion in human breast milk: principles,

pharmacokinetics, and projected consequences, Clin. Pharmacokinet. **5:**1, 1980.

93. Avery, M.E., Does delivery by section matter to the infant? N. Eng. J. Med. **285:**917, 1971.

94. Kafka, H., Hibbard, L.T., and Spears, R.L.: Perinatal mortality associated with cesarean section, Am. J. Obstet. Gynecol. **105:**593, 1969.

95. Greater survival of LBW infants may cause rise in palsy rate, Ob. Gyn. News **15:**1, 1980.

96. Visual, CNS defects high in infants smaller than 1,000 G., Ob. Gyn. News **16:**1, 1981.

97. Young, D., and Mahan, C.: Unnecessary cesareans: ways to avoid them, Minneapolis, 1980, International Childbirth Education Association.

98. Bradley, C.: The effects of hospital experience on postpartum feelings and attitudes of women, doctoral dissertation, Vancouver, B.C., 1976, University of British Columbia.

99. Joy, L.A.: Ramifications of caesarean versus vaginal delivery for the development of maternal attachment, Paper presented at the meeting of the Society for Research in Child Development, San Francisco, March 1979.

100. Affonso, D., and Stichler, J.: Exploratory study of women's reactions to having a cesarean birth, Birth Fam. J. **5:**88, 1978.

101. Doering, S.G.: Unnecessary cesareans: doctor's choice, parent's dilemma. In Stewart, D., and Stewart, L., eds.: Compulsory hospitalization: freedom of choice in childbirth? vol. 1, Marble Hill, Mo., 1979, NAPSAC Reproductions.

102. Cragin, E.B.: Conservation in obstetrics, N. Y. J. Med. **104:**1, 1916.

103. The most popular type of cesarean is a low, horizontal uterine incision. A very strong scar results from these "low, transverse" incisions, so that the risk of uterine rupture during subsequent labor is correspondingly low (0.5%). The direction of the scar on the skin is not necessarily the same as the direction of the scar on the uterus.

104. Golan, A., Sandbank, O., and Rubin, A.: Rupture of the pregnant uterus, Obstet. Gynecol. **56:**549, 1980.

105. Repeat cesarean should not be routine, Ob. Gyn. News **17**(8):16, 1982.

106. Hornbrook, M.: Personal communication, National Center for Health Services Research, Washington, D.C.

107. Horowitz, S.: Personal communication, Health Service Data Dept., Blue Cross & Blue Shield, Jacksonville, Fla. Blue Cross/Blue Shield reports that national figures are not available.

108. Accounting Officer: Personal communication, Shands Teaching Hospital, Gainesville, Fla.

109. March of Dimes Maternal/Newborn Advocate **9**(2):1982.

110. Corea, G.: The cesarean epidemic: who's having this baby, anyway—you or the doctor? Mother Jones, p. 33, July 1980.

111. 23,963 Ob. Gyns. in practice at the end of 1978, Ob. Gyn. News **15:**2, 1980. The Department of Health and Human Services predicts for the medical profession as a whole a surplus of 50% more than needed by the year 2000.

112. Predicted glut of Ob. Gyns. will be good news to some areas, Ob. Gyn. News **16:**1, 1981.

113. 10,000 surplus is expected in Ob. Gyn. by end of decade, Ob. Gyn. News **15:**1980.

114. Haug, J.N., and Kuntzman, K.: Socio-economic factbook for surgery, Chicago, 1980, American College of Surgeons.

115. This average is based on fees for senior and assistant surgeons and anesthesi-

ologists. Most third-party billings for cesarean sections include this medical trio.

116. Review of practice shows "surprising" rise in cesareans, Ob. Gyn. News **14**(1):1, 1979.

117. Owens, A., Earnings: where do you fit in? Med. Econom. **59**:246, 1982.

118. Physician surplus will increase health care cost, Ob. Gyn. News **17**(14):16, 1982.

119. Vayda, E.: A comparison of surgical rates in Canada and in England and Wales, N. Engl. J. Med. **289**(23):1224, 1973.

120. Are primary cesarean section rates too high? Ob. Gyn. News **16**(22):38, 1981.

121. Oakley, A.: Cross-cultural practices. In Chard, T., and Richards, M., eds.: Benefits and hazards of the new obstetrics, Clin. Dev. Med. **64**:18, 1977.

122. Maternal-infant bonding failure can cause depression, Ob. Gyn. News **16**(11): 25, 1981.

123. Letter to NAPSAC from E. and J. M., Reprinted with permission from NAPSAC News **5**(3):21, 1980.

124. Letter to NAPSAC from L. M., Reprinted with permission from NAPSAC News **6**(2):18, 1980.

125. Letter to NAPSAC from Karen Johnston, Reprinted with permission from NAPSAC News **6**(4):17, 1981.

126. The feelings are not unlike those experienced by rape victims, according to some clinicians.

127. Enkin, M.: What happens to normal childbirth in a hospital? influence of advanced technology, NAPSAC News **3**:5, 1978.

128. Rice, R.D.: Maternal-infant bonding: the profound long-term benefits of immediate, continuous skin and eye contact at birth. In Stewart, D., and Stewart, L., eds.: 21st century obstetrics now!, vol. 1, Marble Hill, Mo., 1977, NAPSAC Reproductions.

129. Kennell, J.H., Voos, D.K., and Klaus, M.H.: Parent-infant bonding. In Osofsky, J.D., ed.: Handbook of infant development, New York, 1979, John Wiley & Sons, Inc.

130. Evaluating benefits and risks of obstetric practices—more coordinated federal and private efforts needed, Report to the Congress of the United States by the Comptroller General, Washington, D.C., September 24, 1979, General Accounting Office HRD-79-85.

131. 13 years later—parents learn child is not their son, Tampa Tribune, p. 1, November 28, 1980.

132. Moore, T.D., ed.: Iatrogenic problems in neonatal intensive care, Ross Laboratories, 1976, Columbus, Ohio.

133. Hazuka, B.: Prevention of infection in the nursery, Nurs. Clin. N. Am. **15**(4):825, 1980.

134. Albert, R.K., and Condie, F.: Hand-washing patterns in medical intensive-care units, N. Engl. J. Med. **304**:1465, 1981.

135. Physicians' indifference to accepted sanitary measures may be matched by their indifference to other accepted public health measures. The recognized need for all health personnel in contact with pregnant women to be immunized against rubella far exceeds their willingness to be immunized. Recent studies found that of all categories of health professionals, physicians known to be susceptible to rubella had the lowest rate of participation (22%) in a voluntary rubella immunization program. The studies were prompted by recent outbreaks of rubella in hospital employees, as well as pregnant women. (Ob. Gyn. staff found to need rubella shots, Ob. Gyn. News **16**:1, 1981.)

Chapter 2

1. Health care costs hit $287 billion in 1981, Pharm. Weekly **21**(30):121, 1982.
2. National Prescription Audit, ed. 19, Fort. Washington, Pa., 1980, IMS Press.
3. OTC review helps spur nonprescription drug market, Am. Pharm., **NS22**(10):19, 1982.
4. Is fetal monitoring safe? Washington Post, p. 3, April 16, 1978.
5. Goodlin, R.C., and Haesslein, H.C.: When is it fetal distress? Am. J. Obstet. Gynecol. **128**(4):445, 1977.
6. Marieskind, H.I.: An evaluation of caesarean section in the United States, Final report submitted to U.S. Department of Health, Education and Welfare, 1979, 311–234/4 1–3, p. 63, Washington, D.C., 1980, U.S. Government Printing Office.
7. The 1933 White House Conference on Maternal and Child Health recommended that physicians charge no more for cesarean delivery than for vaginal delivery to avoid charges that money motivates an obstetrician to deliver patients surgically rather than normally. The recommendation was repeated in the government's 1980 survey of factors contributing to the rising cesarean rate. The recommendation has gone unheeded.
8. Haug, J.N., and Kuntzman, K.: Socio-economic factbook for surgery: 1980, Chicago, 1908, American College of Surgeons.
9. Chard, T., and Richards, M., eds.: Benefits and hazards of the new obstetrics, Clin. Dev. Med. **64**:157, 1977.
10. 10,000 surplus is expected in Ob. Gyn. by end of decade, Ob. Gyn. News **15**(22):1, 1980.
11. Montagu, A.: Social impacts of unnecessary intervention and unnatural surroundings in childbirth. In Stewart, D., and Stewart, L., eds.: 21st century obstetrics now! vol. 2, Marble Hill, Mo., 1977, NAPSAC Reproductions.
12. Dr. Murray Enkin quoted in Elkins, V.H.: The rights of the pregnant parent, New York, 1978, Waxwing Productions.
13. Stewart, D.: The limits of science in childbirth. In Stewart, D., and Stewart, L., eds.: 21st century obstetrics now! vol. 2, Marble Hill, Mo. 1977, NAPSAC Reproductions.
14. Oakley, A.: Cross-cultural practices. In Chard, T., and Richards, M., eds.: Benefits and hazards of the new obstetrics, Philadelphia, 1977, J.B. Lippincott Co.
15. Cetrulo, C.L., and Freeman, R.K.: Problems and risks of fetal monitoring. In Aladjem, S., ed.: Risks in the practice of modern obstetrics, St. Louis, 1975, The C.V. Mosby Co.

Chapter 3

1. Lubic, R.W.: Evaluation of an out-of-hospital maternity center for low-risk patients. In Aiken, L.H., ed.: Health policy and nursing practice, New York, 1980, McGraw-Hill Book Co.
2. Ernst, E.K.M., and Lubic, R.W.: Establishing a free-standing birth center, Workshop presentation, Buffalo, June 25, 1983.
3. Editorial, CBCN News **1**:1, 1981. This newsletter was the first for the Cooperative Birth Center Network, now renamed the National Association of Childbearing Centers.
4. Information for establishing standards or regulations for free standing birth centers, CBCN News **1**:3, Feb./May, 1982.

5. American Public Health Association: Policy statement: guidelines for licensing and regulating birth centers, Am. J. Public Health **73**:332, 1983.
6. American College of Obstetricians and Gynecologists, Executive Board: Alternative birth centers, Washington, D.C., Dec. 3–4, 1982, The College.
7. Institute of Medicine and National Research Council: Research issues in the assessment of birth settings, Washington, D.C., 1982, National Academy Press.
8. American Academy of Pediatrics and American College of Obstetricians and Gynecologists: Guidelines for perinatal care, Evanston, Ill., and Washington, D.C., 1983, p. 59. These guidelines for maternal and newborn care represent a collaborative effort by obstetric and pediatric committees and consultants from both organizations.
9. Editorial, CBCN News **1**:2, Summer, 1983.
10. De Vries, R.G.: The alternative birth center: option or cooptation? Women Health **5**:47, Fall, 1980. This article describes findings from a study of 25 inhospital birthing rooms and alternative birth units, not freestanding birth centers.
11. Newton, N., Peeler, D., and Newton, M.: Effect of disturbance on labor, Am. J. Obstet. Gynecol. **101**:1096, 1968.
12. Lubic, R.W., and Ernst, E.K.M. The childbearing center: an alternative to conventional care, Nurs. Outlook **26**:754, 1978.
13. Bennetts, A., and Lubic, R.W.: The free-standing birth centre, Lancet p. 378, February 13, 1982.
14. Network surveys birth centers, CBCN News **1**:4, Summer, 1983.
15. Nielsen, I.: Nurse-midwifery in an alternative birth center, Birth Fam. J. **4**:24, Spring, 1977.
16. Reinke, C.: Outcomes of the first 527 births at The Birthplace in Seattle, Birth **9**:231, Winter, 1982.
17. Lubic, R.W.: Debate: where to give birth. II. Birth center, Childbirth Educ. **2**:32, Summer 1983. The Childbearing Center in New York City charges $1325 with $50 reduction if the fee is paid by the second prenatal visit. A normal delivery in a New York City hospital plus obstetrician fees, on the other hand, costs $3000 or more.
18. Ma Bell gives ok to Birth Center heading in Yellow Pages, CBCN News **1**:1, Summer, 1983.

Chapter 4

1. Stewart, D., Home: the traditional safe place for birth. In Stewart, D., ed.: The five standards for safe childbearing, Marble Hill, Mo., 1981, NAPSAC Reproductions.
2. Brackbill, Y., Woodward, L., McManus, K., and Ireson, M.: Characteristics and medication decisions of women choosing nontraditional birth alternatives, J. Nurse-Midwifery, 1984.
3. Burnett, C.A., and others: Home delivery and neonatal mortality in North Carolina, J.A.M.A. **244**:2741, 1980.
4. Mehl, L.E.: Research on alternatives in childbirth: what can it tell us about hospital practice? In Stewart, D., and Stewart, L., eds.: 21st century obstetrics now! vol. 1, Marble Hill, Mo., 1977, NAPSAC Reproductions.
5. Are primary cesarean section rates too high? Ob. Gyn. News **16**(22):38, 1981.
6. Rubin, G., and others: The risk of childbearing re-evaluated, Am. J. Public Health **71**:712, 1981.

7. Speckhard, M.E.: Maternal mortality surveillance in Puerto Rico. Presented at the 30th Annual ELS Conference, Atlanta, Georgia, April 26, 1981.
8. Cates, W.: Personal communication, Centers for Disease Control, Atlanta, Ga.
9. Barno, A., and others: Minnesota maternal mortality study: five-year general summary, 1950–1954, Obstet. Gynecol. **34:**337, 1957.
10. Mormol, J.G., and others: After office hours: history of the maternal mortality study committees in the United States, Obstet. Gynecol. **34:**133, 1969.

Chapter 5

1. Preston, T.: The clay pedestal, Seattle, 1981, Madrona Publishers, Inc.
2. Enkin, M.W.: LaLeche League Conference, Toronto, July, 1977.
3. McManus, K., and others: Consumer information about prenatal and obstetric drugs, Women Health **7**(1):15, 1982.
4. Following the death at the FDA of the direct, nonoptional, pharmacist-to-consumer drug information program in 1982, the American Medical Association (AMA) launched an indirect, voluntary program of patient medication instruction (the "PMI program"). Under this program, the AMA provides requesting physicians with pads of two-page sheets providing drug information on a particular drug or class of drugs. Information on 20 drugs or drug classes is currently available, with plans for information on 100 more drugs or drug classes in the future. The information sheets are not sent automatically; any physician who wants them must order them and pay for postage and handling. How much drug information will actually trickle down to consumers is still an open question. The AMA plans to evaluate the effectiveness of its program in 1983.
5. Brackbill, Y., McManus, K., and Woodward, L.: Choice of a nontraditional birthplace: home versus birth center, unpublished manuscript, 1982.
6. Mendelsohn, R., Confessions of a medical heretic, Chicago, 1979, Contemporary Books, Inc.
7. Stewart, D.: Informed Consent. In Stewart, D., and Stewart, L., eds.: Compulsory hospitalization: freedom of choice in childbirth? vol. 3, Marble Hill, Mo., 1979, NAPSAC Reproductions.
8. Private medical schools may also let you use their libraries. Practice varies. Ask the head librarian.
9. At a nearby university, the current charge for a Medline search is 50¢ a minute. The average search takes 8 to 10 minutes.
10. The librarian can also show you how to use the companion publication, "Scientific Citation Index."
11. Filmmakers Library, Inc., 133 E. 58th Street, New York, N.Y. 10022. 212–355–6545.
12. Film studios' plan to lease videocassettes bring big outcry from squeezed retailers, Wall Street Journal, p. 25, January 18, 1982.
13. Aladjem, S., ed.: Risks in the practice of modern obstetrics, ed. 2, St. Louis, 1975, The C.V. Mosby Co.
14. Soto, S.: Unnecessary cesareans: what's a mother to do? Alternative Birth Crisis Coalition News **1**(3):3, 1982. Reprinted with permission.

Chapter 6

1. Annas, G.J.: Childbirth and the law: how to work within old laws, avoid malpractice, and influence new legislation in maternity cases. In Stewart, D.,

and Stewart, L., eds.: 21st century obstetrics now! vol. 2, Marble Hill, Mo., 1977, NAPSAC Reproductions.

2. For further information, write to National Women's Health Network, 224 7th St. N.E., Washington, DC 20003.

3. For example, in *State v Osmus*, 276 P. 2d 469 (Wyo. 1954), the court held that criminal conduct cannot be attributed to *nonfeasant* acts of the mother during labor, even if the child dies.

4. In *State v Shephard*, 124 N.W. 2d 712 (Iowa 1963), the mother was convicted of second-degree murder when she gave birth completely unassisted on a cold bathroom floor, left the child on the floor unattended for several minutes, cut the placenta with scissors, and wrapped the baby and put it in a suitcase, where it was later found dead.

5. *Roe v Wade*, 410 U. S. 113, 35 L. Ed. 2d 147, 93 S. Ct. 705 (1973).

6. *Bowland v Mun. Ct. for Santa Cruz Cty., etc.*, 556 P. 2d 1081 (Cal. 1976).

7. See, for example, *Salazar v St. Vincent Hospital*, 619 P. 2d 826 (N. M. App. 1980).

8. *Tyrrell v City and County of San Francisco*, 138 Cal. Rptr. 504 (Cal. App. 1977).

9. *Reyes v Superior Court*, 141 Cal. Rptr. 912 (1977).

10. *Jefferson v Griffin Spalding County Hospital Authority*, 274 S. E. 2d 457 (Ga. 1981).

11. NAPSAC News p. 10, Winter 1981.

12. See, for example, *Raleigh Fitkin-Paul Morgan Mem. Hosp. v Anderson*, 201 A. 2d 537 (N.J. 1964) and *Hoener v Bertinato*, 171 A. 2d 140 (N.J. 1961).

13. For a discussion of parents' rights versus professional rights in the determination of medical care, see Obstet. Gynecol. **58**(2):209, 1981.

14. Alliance for Perinatal Research and Services, Inc.: The Federal monitor, Alexandria, Va., **3**:3, Oct. 20, 1980.

15. Alliance for Perinatal Research and Services, Inc.: The Federal Monitor, Alexandria, Va., **3**:2, Dec. 31, 1980.

16. Stewart, D.: Home: the traditional safe place for birth. In Stewart, D., ed.: The five standards for safe childbearing, Marble Hill, Mo., 1981, NAPSAC Reproductions.

17. *H.R.S. v Carolle Baya*, Circ. Ct., St. John's Co., 79–313 CA (Oct. 1979).

18. Midwifery Practices Act, *Fla. Stat.* § 485.001–485.023 (1982).

19. New West, Mothers and Outlaws p. 81, Dec. 22, 1980.

20. Alliance for Perinatal Research and Services, Inc.: The Federal Monitor, Alexandria, Va., **3**:4, June 1980.

21. Young, D.: Changing childbirth: family birth in the hospital, Rochester, N.Y., 1982, Childbirth Graphics, Ltd.

22. *Campbell v Mincey*, 413 F. Supp. 16 (N.D. Miss. 1975) aff'd. 542 F. 2d 573.

23. NAPSAC News p. 19, Winter 1982.

23a. 42 U.S.C. § 1396(d).

24. American Academy of Pediatrics: Standards and recommendations for hospital care of newborn infants, ed. 6, Evanston, Ill., 1977, The Academy.

25. NAPSAC News pp. 1–2, Spring 1981.

26. Gaskin, I.M.: Spiritual midwifery, Summertown, Tenn., 1978, The Book Publishing Co.

27. Newsweek, p. 79, March 2, 1981.

28. Annas, G.J.: The emerging stowaway: parents' rights in the 1980s, Law Med. Health Care, **10**:32, 1981.

29. *Baier v Woman's Hospital Foundation*, 340 So. 2d 360 (La. App. 1977).

30. *Hulit v St. Vincent's Hospital*, 520, P. 2d 99 (Mont. 1974).
31. *Fitzgerald v Porter Memorial Hospital*, 523 F. 2d 716 (7th Cir. 1975).
32. *Henry v Bronx Lebanon Medical Center*, 385 N.Y.S. 2d. 772, 775 (N.Y. App. 1976).
33. In *Patterson v Van Wiel*, 570 P. 2d 931 (N.M. App. 1977), a maternity patient refused to sign an anesthetic consent form on entering the hospital for delivery. A court determined that consent had been obtained, however, after an anesthetist testified that she agreed to it during labor, although she had no memory of labor.
34. *Lawson v G.D. Searle & Company*, 356 N.E. 2d 779, 783 (Ill. 1976).
35. Stewart, R.B., Cluff, L.E., and Philp, J.R., eds.: Drug monitoring: a requirement for responsible drug use, Baltimore, 1977, Williams & Wilkins.
36. Alliance for Perinatal Research and Services, Inc.: The Federal Monitor, Alexandria, Va. p. 2, Dec. 31, 1979.
37. Alliance for Perinatal Research and Services, Inc.: The Federal Monitor, Alexandria, Va., pp. 1–2, June 21, 1979.
38. Alliance for Perinatal Research and Services, Inc.: The Federal Monitor, Alexandria, Va., **3**:4, May 15, 1983.
39. *Mulder v Parke Davis & Co.*, 181 N.W. 2d 882 (Minn. 1970).
40. Ob-Gyn News **18**(4):23, 1983.
41. Alliance for Perinatal Research and Services, Inc.: The Federal Monitor, Alexandria, Va., Aug. 20, 1979.
42. Women's News Service: Spokeswoman, Falls Church, Va., March 1981, p. 6, The Service.
43. For example, *Fla. Stat.* § 395.202 (1981), which provides in pertinent part that a licensed hospital on request shall furnish to a patient after discharge a copy of all records in the possession of the hospital except those records of a psychiatric nature. In addition, the hospital must allow the individual to examine the original records in the hospital's possession during a reasonable time and in a reasonable manner.
44. Unborn children are not considered persons for *wrongful death statute*.
45. Appeals court construed wrongful death statute as allowing wrongful death action for unborn person.
46. The following cases are examples of courts tolling the statute of limitations because of fraudulent concealment by a physician of the causes of injury: *Tetstone v Adams*, 373 So. 2d 362 (Fla. App 1979); *Lynch v Rubacky*, 424 A. 2d 1169 (N.J. 1981); and *Garcia v Presbyterian Hosp. Ctr.*, 593 P. 2d 487, (N.M. Ct. App. 1979).
47. *Moos v U.S.*, 225 F. 2d 705 (8th Cir. 1955).
48. In *Hively v Higgs*, 253 P. 363 (Or. 1927), a trespass action was successfully brought when a patient consented to an operation on the septum of her nose, but, instead, the physician removed her tonsils.
49. The Court in *Abril v Syntex Laboratories*, Inc. 364 N.Y.S. 2d. 281 (N.Y. 1975), held, however, that since surgical procedures were not involved, the action would be governed by traditional concepts of malpractice and not an assault theory.
50. *Stewart v Rudner*, 84 N.W. 2d 816 (Mich. 1957).
51. The court in *Stewart v Rudner* found that the plaintiff was entitled to recover for pain and suffering and loss of wages directly resulting from the physician's failure to perform a cesarean section as contracted.
52. *Bolden v John Hancock*, 422 F. Supp. 28 (E.D. Mich., 1976).
53. In *Jackson v Anderson*, 230 So. 2d 503 (Fla. App. 1970), the court rejected a

physician's contention that the normal birth of a healthy child precluded suit on policy grounds.

54. 72 CJS Supp. 4 § 2 Products Liability.
55. 402A Restatement of Torts 2d.
56. In Re A.H. Robins Co., Inc., "Dalkon Shield" IUD Products Liability Litigation, 406 F. Supp. 540 (J.P.M.D.L. 1975). The federal appeals court reversed the lower court's class certification in 1982. In re *Northern Dist. of Cal., Dalkon Shield, etc., v A.H. Robins Co., Inc.,* 693 F. 2d 847 (9th Circuit 1982), cert. denied on January 24, 1983, at 103 S.Ct. 817, and the United States Supreme Court would not take the case for consideration.
57. *Jorgensen v Meade Johson Laboratories, Inc.,* 483 F. 2d 237 (10th Circuit 1973).
58. Diethylstilbestrol: Extension of Federal Class Action Procedures to Generic Drug Litigation, 14 University of San Francisco L.R., pp. 461, 464, Spring 1980.
59. 460 F. Supp. 713 (N.D. Ill. 1978).
60. Reference deleted in proof.
61. *Sindell v Abbott Laboratories,* 607 P. 2d 924, (Cal. 1980).
62. The National Law Journal, p. 12, April 6, 1981.
63. 61 Am. Jur. 2d, Physicians and Surgeons, § 369.
64. *Mewherter v Hotter,* 42 Iowa 288 (1875).
65. Prosser, W.: Torts, ed. 4, 1971, St. Paul, West Publishing Co.
66. The trend is not to allow a child to recover for the loss of care by the parents. *Meredith v Scruggs,* 244 F. 2d 604 (9th Cir. 1957). However, courts are beginning to recognize the inherent logic of granting a child the right to recover damages against a third party who has caused injury to a parent: § 69 A.L.R. 3d 528 4.; *Ferriter v Daniel O'Connell's Sons, Inc.,* 413 N.E. 2d 690 (Mass. 1980); *Berger v Weber,* 303 N.W. 2d 424 (Mich. 1981).
67. In *Shockly v Prier,* 225 N.W. 2d 495 (Wis. 1975), the parents of a minor child were allowed to recover for loss of the child's aid, comfort, society, and companionship that resulted from the injuries caused by a physician's negligence. Similarly, in *Drayton v Jiffee Chemical Corp.,* 395 F. Supp. 1081 (N.D. Ohio 1975), a mother was allowed to recover for loss of the child's services and society that resulted from a breach of a manufacturer's express and implied warranties.
68. 25 C.J.S., Damages § 2.
69. 61 Am. Jur. 2d, Physicians and Surgeons, § 218, 329.
70. *Wentling v Jenny,* 293 N.W. 2d 76 (Neb. 1980).
71. *Morrison v MacNamara,* 407 A. 2d 555 (D.C. App. 1979).
72. Vogel, J., and Delgado, R.: To tell the truth: physicians' duty to disclose medical mistakes, 28 U.C.L.A.L.R. 52 (1980).
73. 37 ALR 2d 1284 Hospital Liability.
74. See, for example, *Badeaux v East Jefferson General Hospital,* 364 So. 2d 1348 (La. App. 1978).
75. *Adamski v Tacoma General Hospital,* 579 P. 2d 970 (Wash. App. 1978).
76. Alsobrook, H.B.: Hospital liability and risk management, New York, 1980, New York Practicing Law Institute.
77. 61 Am. Jur 2d, Physicians and Surgeons, § 201.
78. 57 Am. Jur 2d, Negligence, §1.
79. *Vanji v Alhadeff,* New York Queens Co. Sup. Ct., No. 14043, 1975.
80. *Lopez v Beth Israel Hosp.,* Docket No. 16949/74 (Bronx Co. Sup. Ct., N.Y., June 14, 1979).

81. *Yocum v Sutter Mem. Hosp.*, Sacramento Cty. Super. Ct. No. 254 046, (1979), 22 ATLA L., Rep. 329 (1979).

82. Ill. 1980, Sangamon Co., Circ. Ct., No. 250–75.

83. *Madrid v Phelps−Dodge Corp.*, Ariz. Superior Ct., Pima Co., 15–8601, Sept. 7, 1977.

84. *Wale v Barnes*, 278 So. 2d 601 (Fla. 1973).

85. *Schreiber v Cestari and Carpineto*, 338 N.Y.S. 2d 972 (1972).

86. In *Molien v Kaiser Foundation Hospitals*, 616 P. 2d 813 (Cal. 1980), a husband successfully brought an action for the misdiagnosis of syphilis, which ultimately led to divorce. He was allowed to sue for loss of marital consortium and emotional distress.

87. In *Johnson v State*, 334 N.E. 2d 590 (N.Y. 1975), the plaintiff was allowed to recover for emotional distress after being falsely advised that her mother had died. The court allowed recovery based on the fact that the plaintiff's emotional distress had been accompanied by objective physical manifestations.

88. *Deutsch v Shein*, 597 S.W. 2d 141 (Ky. 1980).

89. In *Graf v Taggert*, 204 A. 2d 140 (N.J. 1964), the plaintiff was allowed to recover for emotional upset accompanying childbirth. In *Carter v Public Service Coord. Transport*, 136 A. 2d 15 (N.J. Super. 1957), the plaintiff was entitled to damages for anxiety over possible loss of unborn child where she also sustained personal injury.

90. In *Friel v Vineland Obstetrical and Gynecological Prof. Assoc.*, 400 A. 2d at 147, 149 (N.J. Super. 1979), the court refused to dismiss the action for malpractice even though the plaintiff had failed to produce expert testimony.

91. *Lewis v Read*, 193 A. 2d 255 (N.J. App. 1963).

92. *Hiatt v Groce*, 523 P. 2d 320 (Kan. 1974).

93. U.S. Department of Health and Human Services, Public Health Service, National Institutes of Health: Draft report of the task force on cesarean childbirth, Washington, D.C., 1980, U.S. Government Printing Office.

94. *Henry v Bronx*, 385 N.Y.S. 2d 772, 775 (1976).

95. POF, OB Mal. 665, p. 243.

96. *Rotan v Greenbaum*, 273 F. 2d 830 (D.C. Cir. 1959).

97. See, for example, *Hasemeier v Smith*, 361 S.W. 2d 697 (Mo. 1962).

98. *Troppi v Scarf*, 187 N.W. 2d 511 (Mich. App. 1971).

99. *Speck v Finegold*, 408 A. 2d 496 (Pa. Super. 1979).

100. *Berman v Allan*, 404 A. 2d 8 (N.J. 1979).

101. *Gleitman v Cosgrove*, 227 A. 2d 689 (N.J. 1967).

102. For a comprehensive article on the doctrine of informed consent, see President's Commission for the Study of Ethical Problems in Medicine, Biomedical, and Behavioral Research: Making health care decisions: a report on the ethical and legal implications of informed consent in the patient-practitioner relationship, vol. 3, Washington, D.C., 1982, The Commission.

103. Meisel, A.: The exceptions to the informed consent doctrine: striking a balance between competing values in medical decision-making, Wis. L. Rev., pp. 413–488, 1979.

104. Biklen, D.P., and others: Legislative and social issues committee consent handbook, Washington, D.C., 1977, American Association on Mental Deficiency.

105. Beecher, H.K.: Some guiding principles for clinical investigation, J.A.M.A. **195:**1135, 1966.

106. Bricklin, M.: Male doctors, female patients: can this marriage be saved? Prevention p. 26, February 1981.

107. Annas, G.J.: Rights of hospital patients, New York, 1975, Avon Books.
108. Armitage, K.J., Schneiderman, L.J., and Bass, R.A.: Response of physicians to medical complaints in men and women, J.A.M.A. **241**:2186, 1979.
109. Sparrow, L.: An open letter to the OB Department at Beth Israel Hospital, Boston, Reprinted with permission from NAPSAC News **7**(2):17, 1982.
110. *Downer v Veilleux*, 322 A. 2d 82 (Me. 1974).
111. *Parker v St. Paul*, 335 So. 2d 725 (La. App. 1976).
112. *Charley v Cameron*, 528 P. 2d 1205 (Kan. 1974).
113. *Wale v Barnes*, 278 So. 2d 601 (Fla. 1973).
114. 136 F. Supp. 187 (D.C. La. 1955), aff'd 234 F. 2d 811 (5th Cir.).
115. *Sard v Hardy*, 379 A. 2d 1014 (Md. App. 1977). This case provides an excellent discussion of the doctrine of informed consent.
116. Law, S., and Pan, S.: Pain and profit: the politics of malpractice 113 (1978). Cited in Meisel, A., and Kabnick, L.: Informed consent to medical treatment: an analysis of recent legislation, 41 U. of Pitt. L.R. 407, 419, 1980.
117. Ob-Gyn News **18**:8, 1983.
118. Gavison, R.: Privacy and the limits of the law, 89 Yale L.J. 421, 449, 1980.
119. Legal Advisors Committee: Concern for dying, Am. J. Public Health **73**:918, 1983.
120. Pocinki, L.S., Dogger, S.J., and Schwartz, B.P.: The incidence of iatrogenic injuries: report of the secretary's commission on medical malpractice, Washington, D.C., U.S. Government Printing Office.
121. For an extensive discussion of hospital-acquired infections and facts of numerous cases, see Wenzel, R.P.: CRC handbook of hospital acquired infections, Cleveland, CRC Press.

Chapter 7

1. Young, D.: Changing childbirth: family birth in the hospital, Rochester, N.Y., 1982, Childbirth Graphics, Ltd. This book provides documentation about birth options and strategies to implement them.
2. Stewart, D., and Stewart, L., eds.: The childbirth activists' handbook, Marble Hill, Mo., 1983, NAPSAC Reproductions.
3. Haire, D.: The cultural warping of childbirth, a special report, Minneapolis, 1972, International Childbirth Education Association.
4. Shaw, N.S.: Forced labor: maternity care in the United States, New York, 1974, Pergamon Press, Inc.
5. Arms, S.: Immaculate deception: a new look at women and childbirth in America, Boston, 1975, Houghton Mifflin Co.
6. The Boston Women's Health Book Collective: Our bodies, ourselves: a book by and for women, New York, 1978, Random House, Inc.
7. Klaus, M.H., and Kennell, J.H.: Parent-infant bonding, St. Louis, 1982, The C.V. Mosby Co.
8. Brazelton, T.B.: Behavioral competence of the newborn infant. In Taylor, P.M., ed.: Parent-infant relationships, New York, 1980, Grune & Stratton.
9. International Childbirth Education Association: Position paper on planning comprehensive maternal and newborn services for the childbearing year, Minneapolis, 1979, The Association.
10. Interprofessional Task Force on Health Care of Women and Children: Joint position statement on the development of family-centered maternity/newborn care in hospitals, Chicago, 1978, American College of Obstetricians and Gynecologists.

11. American Public Health Association: Position paper: alternatives in maternity care, Am. J. Public Health **70:**310, 1980.

12. Department of Obstetrics and Gynecology, McMaster University: Family-centered maternity care, Bull. Soc. Obstet. Gynecol. Can. **11**(3):1, 1981.

13. Chard, T., and Richards, M., eds.: Benefits and hazards of the new obstetrics, Philadelphia, 1977, J.B. Lippincott Co.

14. Young, D., ed.: Obstetrical intervention and technology in the 1980s, New York, 1983, The Haworth Press, Inc.

15. Placek, P.J., Taffel, S., and Moien, M.: Cesarean section delivery rates, United States, 1981, Am. J. Public Health **73:**861, 1983.

16. O'Driscoll, K.: Managing dystocia in the primipara, Contemp. Obstet. Gynecol. **19:**193, 1982. Additional features of the "active management" at National Maternity Hospital in Dublin include accurate determination of when labor has begun, stringent patient selection, and constant, one-to-one nursing attendance. If cervical dilatation is below acceptable levels, membranes are ruptured after 1 hour of labor and oxytocin given after 2 hours. At this hospital, 9000 women give birth annually, and the cesarean section rate is less than 5%.

17. Moore, K.: Obstetrician quits rather than live with attorney looking over his shoulder, Houston Chronicle, p. 6, Sept. 18, 1983.

18. Cost of obstetric care is linked to insurance, New York Times, Sept. 11, 1983.

19. Drummond, H.: Over-preventative medicine: how doctors and lawyers are making mountains out of moles, Mother Jones, pp. 12–27, May 1983.

20. DeVries, R.G.: The alternative birth center: option or cooptation? Women Health **5:**47, Fall 1980. It is important to note that this author is discussing the in-hospital birthing room or center, not freestanding birth centers.

21. Nurse-midwifery: Consumer's freedom of choice. Hearing before the Subcommittee on Oversight and Investigations, 96th Cong., 2nd Sess., Washington, D.C., Dec. 18, 1980, U.S. Government Printing Office.

22. Smith, D.: In our own interest: a handbook for the citizen lobbyist in state legislatures, Seattle, 1979, Madrona Publishers, Inc.

23. Christiansen-Ruffman, L., and Catano, J.: Resistance to consumer participation among health planners: a case study of BONDING's encounters with entrenched ideas and structures. Presented at the Canadian Sociology and Anthropology Association Meeting, June 1–4, 1983. The group BONDING (Better Obstetric and Neonatal Decisions In the New Grace) was formed from a coalition of groups and individuals to have input into plans for the new Grace Maternity Hospital in Halifax, Nova Scotia.

24. Fisher, R., and Ury, W.: Getting to yes, New York, 1983, Penguin Books.

A

Glossary

This glossary is not intended to provide rigorous and complete dictionary definitions. Rather it provides working definitions for the purpose of reading this book. To preserve brevity and avoid redundancy, some of the terms here are defined by the use of other terms also found in the glossary. For more thorough and detailed definitions, the reader should consult a medical or legal dictionary.

abortion Expulsion of an embryo or fetus before it is viable.

abruptio placentae Premature detachment of the placenta.

abscess A body site where pus accumulates.

acidosis A condition of the blood of higher than normal acidity resulting from inadequate supplies of oxygen. In the case of a fetus or newborn baby, if blood pH (a measure of acidity) is less than 7.25, the fetus or newborn is considered to be in a state of some degree of asphyxia.

action Proceedings in a court of law where one party demands enforcement of legal rights against another party.

alternative birth center A homelike delivery setting, in-hospital or out-of-hospital (freestanding), where family-centered forms of maternity care are permitted.

American College of Obstetricians and Gynecologists (ACOG) An organization of certified specialists in obstetrics and gynecology.

amnesic A drug that causes loss of memory, for example, scopolamine.

amniocentesis The obtaining of a sample of amniotic fluid during pregnancy for genetic analysis by puncturing the mother's abdomen and womb with a special needle.

amnion A fluid-filled membrane or sac surrounding the fetus in the womb. Also called "bag of waters."

amniotic fluid A transparent liquid surrounding the fetus within the amnion.

amniotomy Surgical rupture of the amnion, usually by means of a long, sharp instrument inserted through the vagina, to induce labor.

analgesia A state of reduced sensibility to pain.

analgesic A drug that induces analgesia.

analog form Fetal monitors, electrocardiograms, and other electronic measuring devices can produce their information in the form of traced lines that go up and down on paper. These line tracings are referred to as "data in analog form." (See also **digital form**.)

anesthesia Loss of feeling or sensation. General anesthesia implies not only a loss of feeling or sensation but also of consciousness and memory. Regional anesthesia implies a loss of feeling or sensation in a restricted area of the body.

anoxia Oxygen deprivation or lack; insufficient oxygen for body cells to perform normal function.

antacid A substance that counteracts or neutralizes acid.

antibiotic An antibacterial substance of biological origin, for example, penicillin, streptomycin.

antiemetic A drug that prevents or relieves nausea or vomiting.

anus Opening of the rectum through which stool passes.

Apgar score An evaluation of five factors in the newborn infant—color, pulse, reflexes, activity, and respiration—made at 1 and 5 minutes after birth. Two points are possible for each factor; thus an infant in the best possible condition would have an Apgar score of 10; 7 to 9 indicates a vigorous infant; 4 to 6 indicates a depressed infant; and 0 to 3 indicates a markedly depressed infant. The rating system was devised by and named after Virginia Apgar, an anesthesiologist.

appellate court A reviewing court; not a trial court or court of first instance. Second level of judicial consideration. Such courts review trial court findings for misapplication of the law to the facts and generally do not question facts as found by the trial court.

asphyxia Suffocation; state of decreased oxygen and increased carbon dioxide in blood and tissues. "Asphyxia neonatorum" is asphyxia in newborns.

aspiration pneumonia Inflammation of the lungs caused by inhalation of foreign substances, such as food or meconium, which usually occurs in mother or fetus during periods of depressed consciousness following obstetrical drug administration.

bag of waters The amnion.

bilirubin A red bile pigment resulting from the normal breakdown of red blood cells. This process may intensify in newborn babies, particularly after administration of certain obstetrical drugs, for example, oxytocin. When increased levels of bilirubin occur in blood tissues (jaundice), the baby's skin appears yellow.

binding Having power to bind or obligate; obligatory.

birth center Usually refers to a freestanding facility, separate from a hospital, where mothers can give birth. (See also **alternative birth center**.)

bonding The spontaneous formation of attachment between mothers and their babies in the period immediately following birth.

Bradley method A method of natural childbirth developed by Robert Bradley, M.D., and promulgated by the American Academy of Husband-Coached Childbirth, which certifies childbirth educators in this method. (See also **Lamaze method**.)

bradycardia Abnormal slowness of heartbeat.

breech presentation The intrauterine position in which the fetus' buttocks or legs ("frank breech") are directly above or in the birth canal.

catheterization A tube passed through a narrow canal into a body part or organ. Urinary catheters pass through the urethra and into the bladder for purpose of draining urine. Catheters are also used in the administration of epidural, saddle block, and caudal anesthesia, in which a puncture wound is made near the mother's spine through which a tube is passed to inject the drugs.

caudal anesthesia A form of regional anesthetic produced by injecting a local anesthetic agent into the end of the spine (*cauda*, Latin for tail).

cause of action An event, a set of facts, or a set of circumstances that give rise to a legally enforceable claim.

cephalopelvic disproportion (CPD) A situation in which the head of the unborn baby is too large to pass through the pelvic bones of the mother.

cerebrovascular accident Brain hemorrhage, blood clot, or stroke.

cervix The lower end of the uterus.

cesarean section The surgical removal of a baby through the mother's abdomen.

childbearing center A freestanding birth center.

class action A means by which one or more members of a class, who share a common interest in the matter at hand, may sue as representative of the entire class for benefit of the entire class.

consideration The inducement to a contract, usually money or the promise to pay money; the cause, motive, price, or impelling influence that induces a contracting party to enter into a contract; the reason or material cause of a contract; a necessary element of a legally enforceable, binding contract.

consortium (loss of consortium) Conjugal fellowship of husband and wife; the legally recognized right of each to the other's company, society, cooperation, affection, and aid. This includes loss or impairment of sexual relations.

contraceptive Any drug, device, or method that prevents conception (union of sperm and egg) or that prevents implantation of a fertilized egg in the uterine wall.

contract A promissory agreement between two or more persons that creates a legal relation that binds the parties to perform their promises.

contraindication Medical "reason" for not applying an intervention. (See also **indication**.)

cord Umbilical cord. The connecting tube between the developing fetus and the placenta through which oxygen, nourishment, and fetal waste pass.

cord prolapse A situation in which the cord delivers before the baby is born.

Demerol A brand name for meperidine, a synthetic narcotic, frequently used as an analgesic in hospital deliveries.

demography The statistical description of a population or group.

dextrose A kind of sugar.

digital form Data produced in numerical form. (See also **analog form**.)

dilation, dilatation Stretching beyond normal dimensions, as the cervix in labor.

discovery rule Generally, the cause of action for medical malpractice will not be held to accrue until the patient knows (or, in exercise of reasonable diligence, should have known) of the alleged malpractice. The discovery rule is important in those cases when the patient discovers the injury after the statute of limitations has elapsed. In these instances, the date of treatment is the date the cause of action became effective.

Doptone A device using the Doppler principle to detect the fetal heartbeat.

Down's syndrome A syndrome of mental retardation resulting from a chromosomal abnormality. The syndrome also includes certain changes in physical features that were commonly thought to be mongolian in nature—hence, the former term "mongolism" for the syndrome.

drug (1) Federal statute: Any article intended for use in diagnosis, cure, mitigation, treatment, or prevention of disease. (2) Random House Unabridged: A chemical substance administered to prevent or cure disease or otherwise enhance physical or mental welfare. (3) Goodman and Gilman, *The Pharmacological Basis of Therapeutics*: Any chemical agent that affects living processes.

dystocia Slow or prolonged labor. (NOTE: The definition of "slow" or "prolonged" is a matter of opinion.)

eclampsia A toxic condition of late pregnancy marked by seizures or convulsions.

elective Done by choice (usually the physician's) rather than by reason of medical need.

elective induction The inducing of labor without medical indication.

electrocardiogram (ECG) A graphic recording of the electrical current produced by the contraction of the heart muscle.

electrode A piece of metal brought into contact with the skin to conduct electrical signals generated by the organism through a wire to an amplifier.

electroencephalogram (EEG) A graphic recording of the electrical fields produced by the action of the brain.

electronic fetal monitor A device that records the fetal heartbeat during labor by means of electrodes attached to or under the baby's scalp.

embryo The fetus in its earliest stages of development (first trimester).

empirical midwife A midwife who acquired her training and skills by apprenticeship and experience rather than in a formal way through structured schooling.

epidural anesthesia or "block" A type of regional anesthesia in which a local anesthetic agent is injected into the epidural space of the spine. (Same as "peridural block" and "extradural block.")

episiotomy Cutting the vulva during childbirth to enlarge the birth opening.

expert testimony Testimony given in relation to some scientific, technical, or professional matter by experts, that is, persons qualified to speak authoritatively by reason of their special training, skill, or familiarity with the subject.

factual settings The actual events, circumstances, and actions that give rise to a cause of action. Once proven or admitted, the law is applied or not applied to such facts to determine each party's legal rights and obligations.

failure to progress See **dystocia.**

family physician A doctor who has undergone special training in family practice. Some family physicians specialize in obstetrics, but such physicians are not the same as "board certified obstetrician/gynecologists." (See also **obstetrician.**)

fecal matter Any excretion of the bowels. (See also **meconium.**)

fetal Concerning the fetus.

fetal distress A situation in which the fetus is partially or completely deprived of oxygen. Obstetrical drugs, fetal monitors, the supine or lithotomy position, and other medical procedures can all contribute to fetal distress.

fetal heart monitor See **electronic fetal monitor.**

fetal monitor See **electronic fetal monitor.**

fetal mortality Stillbirth.

fetus The unborn child during the second and third trimesters.

fiduciary A special relationship between persons because of a trust or confidence placed by one in the other by virtue of the other's special knowledge and training.

filing of such an action The institution of a lawsuit; generally the placement, with the clerk of the court, of a complaint that must also be served on the perceived wrongdoer.

fistula An abnormal connection or channel between two body parts, for example, an opening between the trachea and esophagus.

fontanel, fontanelle Spaces in the skull of the fetus and young infant where the skull bones have not yet grown together.

Food and Drug Administration (FDA) The office of the U.S. government that has authority to approve or disapprove marketing and distribution of various drugs and medical devices and to define their proper scope of use.

forceps An instrument with two blades and handles for forcibly pulling the fetus, by its head, through the birth canal.

freestanding birth center A place, separate from a hospital, where women can give birth with the assistance of professionals and with the availability of appropriate technology for normal births.

general anesthesia Total loss of feeling and sensation, including memory and consciousness. (See also **anesthesia.**)

gestation The average length of gestation, measured from the first day of the last menstrual period, is 280 days or 40 weeks. However, there is considerable individual variation from this figure (even when mistakes and inaccuracies in determining gestational age are set aside), and lengths of gestation from 259 days (37 completed weeks) to 293 days (42 completed weeks) are by international agreement regarded as normal. Babies born within these limits are called "term babies." Babies born earlier are called "preterm babies," and those born later are called "postterm babies." Recent investigations concluded that the limits of normal term should really have been set between 38 and 41 completed weeks instead of between 37 and 42 weeks.

gestational age The age of a fetus from the time of conception; however, because the time of conception is never known with certainty, gestational age is also measured from the first day of the mother's last menstrual period.

granny midwife An empirical midwife who historically represented the majority of midwives in America until the mid-twentieth century. Most granny midwives were older, southern, and black.

hematoma An accumulation of blood, usually clotted, that forms a mass. This is sometimes seen on a newborn baby's head following traumatic delivery.

hemorrhage Excessive bleeding.

high forceps Forceps applied when the baby's head has not yet descended beyond the narrowest passage of the birth canal. (See also **forceps** and **low forceps**.)

high-risk pregnancy A term used to describe the probability that complications of delivery may occur.

home birth When used by home birth advocates, the term refers to a planned, attended birth at home with prenatal care and hospital back-up if needed. When used by home birth opponents, the term is taken to mean all forms of out-of-hospital birth including accidents on the way to the hospital, miscarriages at home, involuntary home births by those too poor to afford the hospital, unattended and unplanned home births, as well as births followed by homicides by unwed mothers who do not want their babies.

hospital birth Any birth taking place in a hospital. The U.S. National Center for Health Statistics, however, also includes births in freestanding birth centers as "hospital births" since, by their way of thinking, both are "institutions."

hyaline membrane disease See **respiratory distress syndrome.**

hypertension High blood pressure.

hypotension Low blood pressure.

hypoxia Oxygen deficiency.

iatrogenic Produced or caused by a physician.

idiopathic Of unknown or obscure cause.

independent contractor One who contracts to do a piece of work according to his or her own methods and is subject to his or her employer's control only as to end product or final result of his or her work; one who is not an employee.

Index Medicus A monthly index of articles from the medical literature, listed by subject and by author. A separate section deals with bibliographies of medical reviews. It serves as the authority for the National Library of Medicine catalogue and for MEDLINE computerized searches. It is a valuable storehouse of information resources.

indication Medical "reason" for applying an intervention. (See also **contraindication.**)

induction of labor The artificial initiation of labor by mechanical or chemical means.

infant mortality Infant deaths per 1000 live births occurring in the first year of life.

injunctive relief An order of the court forbidding the party to whom it is directed from doing some act or permitting servants or agents to perform the act.

intervention In obstetrics, an invasive procedure that literally intervenes or interferes with the natural process of birth. The term denotes active interference and implies meddling with Mother Nature.

intraabdominal Inside the abdomen.

intracranial Within the skull.

intrauterine Within the uterus.

intravenous (IV) Literally, within a vein; a catheter or needle inserted into a blood vessel for the purpose of introducing various fluids and drugs.

jaundice A yellowing of the skin in newborns in the first days of life caused by the presence of bilirubin. (See also **bilirubin**.)

Kegel exercises Voluntary contraction of muscles of a woman's pelvis to improve their strength and tone.

ketamine A general anesthetic drug.

labor Contractions of the uterus resulting in the birth of a baby.

laceration A tear. In childbirth, the perineum can tear. (See also **perineum**.)

Lamaze method A set of distraction techniques, including complex breathing patterns, devised by Fernand Lamaze, M.D., as an alternative to drugs in reducing a woman's awareness of pain in labor. The Lamaze method is promoted by the American Society for Prophylaxis in Obstetrics (ASPO) which certifies childbirth educators in this method. The Lamaze method is not the same as "natural childbirth." (See also **Bradley method**.)

lay midwife An empirical midwife.

legal theory The conceptual result of each party to an action applying the law to the facts of the case. One theory forms a basis for liability, the other theory forms grounds for a defense. Determination by the court of the superior theory decides which party will prevail in the action.

liability A broad legal term encompassing responsibility for almost every character of hazard—absolute, contingent, or likely—that a court will recognize and enforce.

liable (1) Bound or obliged in law or equity. (2) Justly or legally responsible or answerable to another.

lithotomy position Horizontal or supine position. A woman giving birth in this position is flat on her back with legs spread and in stirrups.

litigate To seek relief in a court of law; the act of carrying on a suit in a court of law; hence, any controversy that must be decided on evidence.

local anesthetic A drug administered to a specific region or area of the body to deaden that area to sensation.

low forceps Forceps applied when the baby's head has already descended well into the birth canal.

lower court A court of restricted jurisdiction and subject to review or correction by higher courts; not a court of last resort.

low-risk pregnancy The probability that pregnancy and childbirth will be uncomplicated (uneventful, normal). (See also **high-risk pregnancy**.)

L/S ratio A test to determine fetal lung maturity. A sample is taken of the amniotic fluid by amniocentesis, which is then analyzed for its lecithin (L) and sphingomyelin (S) content. The ratio, L/S, of these two substances is an index of lung maturity. The test is about 80% accurate, but only when combined with other tests.

malpractice, medical Professional misconduct toward a patient; bad, wrong, or injudicious treatment resulting in injury, unnecessary suffering, or death of the patient.

maternal-infant bonding See **bonding**.

maternal mortality Any death of a woman related to pregnancy or to childbirth.

mechanical extraction Delivery by forceps or vacuum extraction.

meconium A baby's first stool. Sometimes this is passed in the womb before birth.

meconium aspiration The inhalation of meconium by the newborn into its lungs.

medication Drug, medicine. See also **drug**.

meperidine See **Demerol.**

mid forceps Forceps applied when the baby has descended midway down the birth canal.

midwife A birth attendant whose basic philosophy is belief in nature and who supports the mother in the natural process of birth. Midwives do a minimum of intervention and usually do not administer drugs or perform surgery. Some do episiotomies. (See also **empirical midwife, lay midwife, granny midwife,** and **nurse-midwife.**)

midwifery A philosophical approach to assisting women in birth that emphasizes support for mothers in giving birth naturally rather than in "delivering babies" and "intervention." The medical model is generally in contradiction to the philosophy of midwifery.

miscarriage The spontaneous expulsion of an embryo or fetus before it is viable (usually about 24 to 28 weeks).

monitor See **electronic fetal monitor.**

morbidity The state of being diseased, injured, or ill.

mortality Death.

mortality rate The number of deaths per 1000 live births (when dealing with fetuses and babies) or the number of deaths per 100,000 pregnancies (when considering mothers).

motion An application made to a court or judge for the purpose of obtaining a rule or order directing something to be done in favor of the applicant. It is usually made within the framework of an existing action or proceeding.

motion for a stay An application to the court requesting a judicial order to stop, refrain, or hold in abeyance some act or action of another.

multipara A woman who has given birth to more than one child.

multiparous Bearing or having borne more than one child.

narcotic Any drug that produces sleep and stupor and, at the same time, relief from pain.

narcotic antagonist A drug whose action tends to cancel that of a narcotic.

natural childbirth An educated approach to childbirth in which one studies the body's natural tendencies and processes and attempts to work in harmony with these forces. Natural childbirth is opposed to such unnatural interventions as drugs and devices.

negligence The omission of conduct that a reasonable and prudent person, guided by the ordinary considerations that regulate human affairs, would do; conduct that a reasonable and prudent person would not do.

neonatal mortality The number of deaths per 1000 live births of babies during the first 28 postpartum days.

neonate (1) Literally, newborn. (2) A baby less than 28 days old.

neonatologist A pediatrician who specializes in newborn babies. (See also **perinatologist**.)

neurologic damage Damage to the nervous system; used principally for damage to the central nervous system or brain.

nonfeasant Nonperformance of some act that ought to be performed or total neglect of duty.

normal (1) Unaffected by disease or experimental treatment. (2) Occurring naturally. (3) Average; mean, middle, or median value; the usual condition, degree, or quantity. NOTE: Definitions of the term "normal" are subject to considerable arbitrariness, change over time, and change with context. It is always advisable to check on the user's particular meaning at the time and in the context used.

nosocomial Caused or produced by a hospital.

nulliparous Never having borne children; used in the United States as a synonym for "primiparous."

nurse-midwife A registered nurse who has taken a formal training program accredited by the American College of Nurse-Midwives (ACNM). All nurse-midwifery training schools are affiliated with a college or university and are usually associated with schools of nursing and/or medicine. (See also **midwife**.)

obstetrician/gynecologist (OB/GYN) A physician who has taken a formal training program and passed prescribed exams accredited by the American Board of Obstetricians and Gynecologists. (See also **family physician**.)

obstetrics That branch of medicine concerned with childbirth and childbearing. Although the term comes directly from the Latin for midwifery, present day obstetrics, with its emphasis on the medical/disease model and technological interventions, is diametrically opposed, both philosophically and practically, to midwifery.

oral contraceptive (OC) "The Pill."

outcome Result, consequence, issue. In childbirth, the outcome is the state of the baby as well as that of the mother.

out-of-hospital birth See **home birth** and **hospital birth**.

oxytocin A drug that causes the uterus to contract. As a uterine stimulant, it is used to induce labor or to accelerate existing labor.

paracervical block The injection of local anesthetic drugs around the cervix to block pain.

parturient (1) A woman in the process of giving birth. (2) Giving birth; pertaining to birth.

parturition The act or process of giving birth.

pediatrician A physician who specializes in the care of children. (See also **neonatologist**.)

pelvic floor The perineal tissues, including pubococcygeus muscle, situated at the bottom of the pelvis.

pelvic relaxation Weakening of the pubococcygeus muscle of the lower pelvis. The cervix may protrude, and there may be decreased inability to control bladder and bowel. This condition can sometimes be caused by episiotomy.

pelvis (From the Latin for *basin*) The basin-shaped ring of bone at the end of the trunk; it supports the spine and is supported by the legs.

perinatal Concerning the period that begins the twentieth to twenty-eighth week of gestation and ends the seventh to twenty-eighth day after birth.

perinatal mortality Death of an infant or fetus during the perinatal period. (See also **perinatal**.)

perinatologist An obstetrician who specializes in newborn babies. (See also **neonatologist**.)

perineum (perineal) The region between the anus and the opening of the vagina.

Pitocin A brand name for oxytocin.

placenta The flat, round organ that, following fertilization of the egg, develops in and attaches to the uterus. It attaches to the fetus by means of the umbilical cord. Together with the cord, it functions to deliver nutrients and oxygen from mother to fetus and waste products from fetus to mother.

placenta previa An abnormal condition in which the placenta becomes positioned over the opening of the womb.

placental abruption See **abruptio placentae**.

placental hemorrhage Abnormal bleeding due to premature separation of the placenta from the inside wall of the womb. In a normal birth, the placenta will naturally separate from the womb after the baby's birth when the womb is in a state of contraction. Upon normal separation of the placenta the connecting blood vessels from the womb are pinched shut and only a small amount of blood is lost.

plaintiff The party who complains or sues in a civil action and is so named on the record; a person who brings an action in a court of law.

postnatal Following childbirth. (Term usually applied to baby.)

postpartum Following childbirth. (Term usually applied to mother.)

postpartum depression Depression of the mother following childbirth, usually due to reactions to drugs received in labor, isolation from family, and other factors. Postpartum depression is common in hospital births but extremely uncommon in home births. This is also called "new baby blues."

preeclampsia Signs in pregnancy that eclampsia may be developing, including abnormalities in blood pressure, protein in the urine, severe edema, and so forth.

premature rupture of membranes (PROM) The spontaneous rupture of the bag of waters without the onset of labor contractions that lead to a birth. The exact definition is arbitrary among health professionals and may vary from 12 hours up to a week.

prematurity See **preterm birth**.

prenatal After conception and before birth.

prenatal risk factors Conditions that decrease the probability of a normal pregnancy and delivery, for example, hypertension, previous miscarriages. (See also **high-risk pregnancy, low-risk pregnancy.**)

presentation The position of the fetus in the uterus at the time of birth; that part of the fetus presenting first through the cervix.

preterm birth Birth of a baby before the completion of 37 weeks of pregnancy. The average length of gestation, measured from the first day of the last menstrual period, is 280 days or 40 weeks. However, there is considerable individual variation concerning this number even when mistakes and inaccuracies in determining gestational age are set aside. Lengths of gestation from 259 days (37 completed weeks) to 293 days (42 completed weeks) are by international agreement regarded as normal. Babies born within these limits are called "term babies." Babies born earlier are called "preterm babies," and those born later are called "postterm babies." Recent investigations lead to the conclusion that the limits of normal term should really have been set between 38 and 41 completed weeks instead of between 37 and 42 weeks.

primipara A woman who has given birth to one child.

primiparous Bearing or having borne only one child.

prolapsed cord See **cord prolapse**.

prophylactic A procedure or intervention done "just in case" with the idea of prevention in mind. For example, episiotomy is a prophylactic procedure done to prevent laceration of the perineum.

pudendal block The injection of local anesthetic around the pudendal nerve to block pain.

reasonable person standard The degree of care an ordinary prudent person would exercise under like circumstances. Failure to exercise such care generally results in a person's being deemed negligent. (See also **standard of care.**)

rectum The lowest part of the large intestine leading to the anus.

regional anesthesia Loss of feeling or sensation in a restricted area of the body.

resistant organism A pathogen that does not respond to the usual modes of treatment.

respiratory distress syndrome (RDS) A complex of symptoms in the newborn including difficulty in breathing, hyaline membranes, cyanosis, and other respiratory problems. The lungs of the newborn do not expand properly because of the presence of hyaline. This disease is associated with prematurity, perinatal asphyxia, maternal diabetes, the second born of twins, and cesarean section. It is also called "idiopathic respiratory distress" and used to be called "hyaline membrane disease."

restraint of trade Contracts or combinations that eliminate competition, effect a monopoly, artificially maintain prices, or otherwise hamper or obstruct the course of trade and commerce as it would be carried on if left to the control of natural economic forces.

Rh isoimmunization Rh-negative mothers bearing Rh-positive children can make an antibody against the Rh-positive red blood cell antigen. This antibody can cross the placenta, destroy the baby's red blood cells, and thereby lead to anemia and even death. The administration of anti-Rh antibody to the mother immediately after birth prevents the subsequent formation of the mother's own antibody and thereby protects future fetuses.

risk See **high-risk pregnancy, low-risk pregnancy, prenatal risk factors.**

saddle block A form of regional anesthesia produced by injecting a local anesthetic agent into the spine; so named because the loss of feeling is in the area of the groin that would be in contact with a saddle if one were riding a horse.

scopolamine A drug that apparently does not reduce the sensation of pain but acts as an amnesic so that the mother forgets having experienced the pain. The use of this drug is now generally condemned by medical schools, but its use continues in many areas of the United States; also called "scope" or "twilight sleep."

sedative A drug that produces a quieting effect.

sedative-hypnotic A drug that produces a quieting effect and sleep.

socioeconomic status A general term referring to one's level of income, standard of living, educational background, and, in some cases, racial and/or cultural status.

sonogram An analog image of the fetus obtained by penetrating the mother's abdomen with ultrasonic sound vibrations that are then reflected back according to the position, shape, and size of the fetus.

spontaneous abortion See **miscarriage.**

standard of care In law of negligence, that degree of care which a reasonably prudent person should exercise under same or similar circumstances. If a person's conduct falls below such standards, he may be liable in damages for injuries or damages resulting from his conduct. In medico-legal malpractice cases, a standard of care is applied to measure the competence of the professional. The traditional standard for doctors is that they exercise the "average degree of skill, care, and diligence exercised by members of the same profession" (from Black's Law Dictionary).

statute A law enacted by the legislative branch of the government.

statute of limitations A period after a cause of action accrues in which an action must be brought before the court. If an action is not brought within this period, no suit will be allowed. See **discovery rule** as to when a cause of action accrues.

stay A suspension of the case or some designated part of it. A stay is a kind of injunction with which a court freezes its proceedings at a particular point.

stillbirth The birth of a dead fetus.

strict liability Liability without fault. Reasonable care, good faith, or ignorance of a defect will not save the defendant. The term is generally applied to manufacturers and sellers of defective or hazardous products.

supine Lying on one's back. (See also **lithotomy position.**)

surgical delivery See **cesarean section.**

tachycardia Abnormally fast heartbeat.

teaching hospital A hospital that is associated with a teaching institution and in which medical and/or nursing students work with patients. Teaching hospitals have higher rates of perinatal and maternal death than nonteaching hospitals.

technological, technology, high-tech In obstetrics, deliveries characterized by the use of interventions. Obstetrics is the technological approach to childbirth (high-tech deliveries).

teratogen An agent that produces anatomical, physiological, or behavioral changes when administered to an organism during the prenatal, perinatal, or postnatal development of its central nervous system.

therapeutic privilege A physician's right to withhold from a patient a diagnosis or contemplated mode of treatment. This right may be exercised only when disclosure of such would substantially increase the risk of emotional harm to the patient.

toll the period (the statute of limitations) Removal of the bar to an action imposed by the passage of time specified in the statute of limitations. Generally granted only on introduction of facts that show just cause for not applying the limitation.

toxemia Symptoms leading to eclampsia. (See **preeclampsia.**)

toxic Poisonous; producing adverse effects.

toxin Any substance causing undesirable or adverse effects in the body.

tranquilizer A drug that reduces fear, anxiety, tension, concern. Examples of tranquilizers frequently used in obstetrics are chlorpromazine (Thorazine), hydroxyzine (Atarax, Vistaril), promazine (Sparine), promethazine (Phenergan), propiomazine (Largon), and triflupromazine (Vesprin).

ultrasonogram See **sonogram.**

ultrasound The high-frequency, mechanical energy used in the production of a sonogram. The safety of this energy and the advisability of its use for fetal assessment have not been evaluated.

umbilical cord See **cord.**

unconstitutional That which is contrary to the constitution; legislation that conflicts with some provision of the United States Constitution.

uterine Pertaining to the uterus.

uterus The sac of muscles in which the fetus develops and that contracts during labor to push the fetus out; also called "womb."

vacuum extractor A suction device affixed to the unborn baby's head to pull the baby out; sometimes called "vacuum forceps."

vagina The canal leading from the womb to the outside of the mother's body.

vaginal examination A medical examination made by inserting the fingers through the vagina to determine such things as the condition of the cervix and the size of the pelvis.

Valium A brand name for diazepam, a tranquilizing drug.

vasoconstrictor/vasopressor An antihypotensive drug causing the blood vessels to constrict. Examples of such drugs used in obstetrics are ephedrine, epinephrine (Adrenalin), mephentermine (Wyamine), metaraminol (Aramine), methoxamine (Vasoxyl), norepinephrine, levarterenol (Levophed), and phenylephrine (Neo-Synephrine).

viable Capable of living. This term is applied to a newborn infant, and especially to one prematurely born, who is born alive and appears to be able to continue living.

vulva The external part of the female genital organs.

waiver The intentional or voluntary relinquishment of a known right or such conduct as warrants an inference of the relinquishment of such right.

womb See **uterus**.

wrongful death action A type of lawsuit brought on behalf of deceased persons' beneficiaries that alleges that death was attributed to the willful or negligent act of another. (From Black's Law Dictionary.)

Appendix

B

Suggested Readings and Films

The books and articles listed may be used to supplement the material presented in this book.

Introduction
Historical Perspectives on Birthing
Corea, G.: The hidden malpractice, New York, 1977, Jove. Chapter 12: Midwives.
Courter, G.: Midwife, Boston, 1981, Houghton Mifflin Co.
Wertz, R.W., and Wertz, D.C.: Lying-in: a history of childbirth in America, New York, 1977, The Free Press.

Chapter 1
Alternative Childbirth
International Childbirth Education Association: Position paper on planning comprehensive maternal and newborn services for the childbearing year, Minneapolis, Minn., September 1979, ICEA.
Romalis, S., ed.: Childbirth: alternatives to medical control, Austin, Tex., 1981, University of Texas Press.
Stewart, D., ed.: The five standards for safe childbearing, Marble Hill, Mo., 1981, NAPSAC Reproductions.
Young, D.: Changing childbirth: family birth in the hospital, Rochester, N.Y., 1982, Childbirth Graphics, Ltd.

Critical Accounts of Medicalized Childbirth
Arms, S.: Immaculate deception, New York, 1975, Bantam Books, Inc.
Corea, G.: The hidden malpractice, New York, 1977, Jove. Chapter 11: Childbirth.
Haire, D.: The cultural warping of childbirth, J. Trop. Pediatr. Environ. Child Health **19:**171–191, 1973.
Harrison, M.: A woman in residence, New York, 1982, Random House, Inc.
Rothman, B.K.: In labor: women and power in the birthplace, New York, 1982, W.W. Norton Co., Inc.
Shaw, N.: Forced labor: maternity care in the United States, vol. 1, Elmsford, N.Y., 1974, Pergamon Press, Inc.

Diet in Pregnancy and Delivery
Brewer, S., and Brewer, T.: What every pregnant woman should know: the truth about diets and drugs in pregnancy, ed. 2, New York, 1979, Penguin Books.

Electronic Fetal Monitoring: Description and Evaluation
Banta, D., and Thacker, S.: Electronic fetal monitoring: is it of benefit? Birth Fam. J. **6**(4):237, 1979.

International Childbirth Education Association: Position statement on electronic fetal monitoring, ICEA News **20**:4, 1981.

Episiotomy
Brendsel, C., Peterson, G., and Mehl, L.E.: Episiotomy: facts, fictions, figures and alternatives. In Stewart, D., and Stewart, L., eds.: Compulsory hospitalization: freedom of choice in childbirth? vol. 1, Marble Hill, Mo., 1979, NAPSAC Reproductions.

Kitzinger, S.: Some women's experiences of episiotomy, London, 1981, National Childbirth Trust.

Popular Reference Sources on Drugs of All Descriptions
Graedon, J.: The people's pharmacy, ed. 2, New York, 1980, Avon Books.

Handbook of nonprescription drugs, ed. 6, Washington, D.C., 1979, American Pharmaceutical Association. Provides information about drug products available to treat minor ailments.

Long, J.: The essential guide to prescription drugs: what you need to know for safe drug use, New York, 1980, Harper & Row Publishers, Inc. Covers much the same ground as *Physician's Desk Reference.*

Physician's desk reference for prescription drugs, Oradell, N.J., 1982, Medical Economics Books. New edition published yearly. Nicknamed "PDR," this reference source contains descriptions of intended use, side effects, etc. of most prescription drugs. The descriptions are written by the manufacturing companies but approved by the FDA. The New York City Public Library reports PDR is the most popular book in their reference section.

Silverman, H.M., and Simon, G.I.: The pill book: the illustrated guide to the most prescribed drugs in the United States, New York, 1979, Bantam Books, Inc.

United States pharmacopeia dispensing information (for patients), Rockville, Md., 1981, The United States Pharmacopeial Convention. Periodic updates. This new reference periodical is intended for the nonprofessional. It is very readable and easily understood. Current coverage is not yet comprehensive, but more drugs are added each year.

Wilson, J.T., and others: Drug excretion in human breast milk: principles, pharmacokinetics, and projected consequences, Clin. Pharmacokinet. **5**:1, 1980. Technical. Unfortunately, no counterpart is available for the interested nonprofessional.

Wolfe, S.M.: Pills that don't work, New York, 1981, Farrar, Straus & Giroux, Inc. Written for consumers by Nader's Health Research Group, this book deals with drug efficacy (effectiveness) rather than safety.

Surgical Delivery
Cohen, N.W., and Estner, L.J.: Silent knife: cesarean prevention and vaginal birth after cesarean, South Hadley, Mass., 1983, J.F. Bergin Publishers, Inc.

Marieskind, H.I.: An evaluation of cesarean section in the United States, Final report submitted to U.S. Department of Health, Education and Welfare, 1979,

311–234/4 1–3, Washington, D.C., 1980, U.S. Government Printing Office. Meant for the professional, but easily understandable by the nonprofessional.

McKay, S., ed.: Vaginal birth following cesarean section, Int. Childbirth Educ. Assoc. Rev. **3**(3/4):1979. Available through International Childbirth Education Association, P.O. Box 20048, Minneapolis, Minn. 55420.

Young, D., and Mahan, C.: Unnecessary cesareans: ways to avoid them, Minneapolis, Minn., 1980, International Childbirth Education Association. Available through International Childbirth Education Association, P.O. Box 20048, Minneapolis, Minn. 55420.

Parent-Infant Bonding

Klaus, M.H., and Kennell, J.H.: Parent-infant bonding, ed. 2, St. Louis, 1982, The C.V. Mosby Co.

Taylor, P.M., ed.: Parent-infant relationships, New York, 1980, Grune & Stratton, Inc.

Chapter 2

The following references deal with general problems in medicine and doctor-patient relationships. None focuses exclusively on childbirth, although issues in childbirth appear frequently as examples.

Blum, R.H., Sadusk, J., and Waterson, R.: The management of the doctor-patient relationship, New York, 1960, McGraw-Hill Book Co.

Burnham, J.C.: American medicine's golden age: what happened to it? Science **215**:1474, 1982.

Harrison, M.: A woman in residence, New York, 1982, Random House, Inc.

Illich, I.: Medical nemesis: the expropriation of health, New York, 1976, Bantam Books, Inc.

Klaw, S.: The great American medicine show, New York, 1976, Penguin Books.

Mendelsohn, R.S.: Confessions of a medical heretic, Chicago, 1979, Contemporary Books, Inc.

Millman, M.: The unkindest cut, New York, 1977, William Morrow & Co., Inc. See also Millman's suggested readings.

Preston, T.: The clay pedestal: a reexamination of the doctor-patient relationship, Seattle, 1981, Madrona Publishers, Inc.

Rushmer, R.: Humanizing health care: alternative futures for medicine, Cambridge, Mass., 1978, The MIT Press. More academic and less critical than other suggested reading.

Starr, P.: The social transformation of American medicine, New York, 1982, Basic Books, Inc.

Stewart, D.: The limits of science in childbirth. In Stewart, D., and Stewart, L., eds.: 21st century obstetrics now! vol. 2, Marble Hill, Mo., 1977, NAPSAC Reproductions.

Chapter 3

As more women have babies in birth centers, doctors, hospitals rethink obstetric procedures, Wall Street Journal, Nov. 29, 1983, p. 60.

Bennetts, A., and Lubic, R.W.: The free-standing birth centre, Lancet, Feb. 13, pp. 378–380, 1982.

Cohen, R.L.: A comparative study of women choosing two different childbirth alternatives, Birth **9**:13–19, Spring, 1982.

Institute of Medicine and National Research Council: Research issues in the assessment of birth settings, Washington, D.C., 1983, National Academy Press.

Lubic, R.W., and Ernst, E.K.M.: The Childbearing Center: an alternative to conventional care, Nursing Outlook **26**:754–760, 1978.

Mather, S.: Women's interests in alternative maternity facilities, J. Nurse-Midwifery **25**:3–11, May/June, 1980.

Nielsen, I.: Nurse-midwifery in an alternative birth center, Birth Family J. **4**:24–27, Spring, 1977.

Reinke, C.: Outcomes of the first 527 births at The Birthplace in Seattle, Birth **9**:231–238, Winter, 1982.

Chapter 4

Why Are Hospital Births Less Safe than Home Births?

Baldwin, R.: Special delivery: the complete guide to informed birth, Millbrae, Calif., 1979, Les Femmes Publishing. This book stresses parental assumption of greater responsibility in any birth setting.

Bean, C.A.: Methods of childbirth, rev. ed. New York, 1982, Doubleday & Co., Inc.

The Boston Women's Health Book Collective: Our bodies, ourselves: a book by and for women, New York, 1977, Simon & Schuster. In this extremely popular book, the sections on pregnancy and delivery are "naturally" oriented.

Bradley, R.: Husband coached childbirth, ed. 3, New York, 1981, Harper & Row Publishers, Inc. This classic stresses the husband/father's role in birthing and the couple's role in decision making.

Brewer, G.S., and Greene, J.P.: Right from the start, Emmaus, Penn., 1981, Rodale Press, Inc. Nontraditional and practical. Covers pregnancy, delivery, and early postnatal periods.

Gaskin, I.M.: Spiritual midwifery, Summertown, Tenn., 1978, The Book Publishing Co. The Farm, America's biggest and most successful cooperative, is famous for its midwifery program. This book, intended for both parents and midwives, is written in down-to-earth terms. It contains lots of illustrations and examples.

Kitzinger, S.: The complete book of pregnancy and childbirth, New York, 1980, Alfred A. Knopf, Inc.

Kitzinger, S., and Davis, J.A., eds.: The place of birth, Oxford, England, 1978, Oxford University Press. A popular British book examines home and hospital as places of birth. It is suitable for parents and professionals alike.

Myles, M.F.: Textbook for midwives, ed. 9, New York, 1981, Churchill Livingstone, Inc.

Stewart, D., ed.: The five standards for safe childbearing, Marble Hill, Mo., 1981, NAPSAC Reproductions. This book and the following one cover a wide variety of childbirth topics. It is published by the International Association of Parents and Professionals for Safe Alternatives in Childbirth (NAPSAC), the country's largest consumer-oriented childbirth organization. Available from NAPSAC Reproductions, P.O. Box 267, Marble Hill, Mo. 63764.

Stewart, D., and Stewart, L., eds.: 21st century obstetrics now! Marble Hill, Mo., 1978, NAPSAC Reproductions.

Stewart, D., and Stewart, L., eds.: Compulsory hospitalization: freedom of choice in childbirth? Marble Hill, Mo., 1979, NAPSAC Reproductions.

White, G.: Emergency childbirth, a guide to handle birth crises, available from NAPSAC Reproductions, P.O. Box 267, Marble Hill, Mo. 63764.

Chapter 5
Information, Decision Making, and Informed Consent

President's Commission for the Study of Ethical Problems in Medicine and Biomedical and Behavioral Research: Making health care decisions: the ethical and
legal implications of informed consent in the patient-practitioner relationship,
3 vols., Washington, D.C., October, 1982, The Commission.

How to Get the Information You Need

Binger, J.L., and Jensen, L.M.: Lippincott's guide to nursing literature, Philadelphia, 1980, J.B. Lippincott Co. This book's purpose is to provide a quick-access
guide to nursing articles and books.

Books in print, New York, latest edition, R.R. Bowker Co. Bookstores as well as libraries carry this comprehensive listing of "trade" books, which are cross-indexed
by author, title, and subject. It also serves as an index to the in-depth material
contained in the Publishers' Trade List Annual.

Chen, C.C.: Health sciences information sources, Cambridge, Mass., 1981, The
MIT Press. Intended as an annotated reference manual for health science professionals and a textbook for library students. Chapters cover health sciences, reference tools, guides to the literature, bibliographies, encyclopedias, dictionaries,
handbooks, statistical sources, atlases, nonprint material, and so forth.

Getting yours: a consumer's guide to obtaining your medical record, Washington,
D.C., 1980, Health Research Group. Updated version of the booklet by Health
Research Group. Gives state-by-state survey of medical record access laws, explanation of how patients in federal facilities can obtain their records, actual
contents of a medical record and how to obtain one's own, and information on
promoting legislation to provide for unrestricted patient access. Available for
$2.50 from Health Research Group, Dept. MR, 2000 P St. N.W., Suite 708, Wash-
ington, D.C. 20036.

Index medicus. Indexes more than 2300 periodicals in medicine, health sciences,
and related fields. Individual articles are cross-indexed by subject matter as well
as by title and authors' names. A separate section covers bibliographies of medical reviews. Index Medicus serves as the authority for the National Library of
Medicine catalogue and for MEDLINE computerized search and retrieval system.

Medical books in print, latest edition, New York, R.R. Bowker Co. Books in medicine and allied fields are indexed by author and title within subject classifica-
tions.

Morton, L.T.: How to use a medical library, ed. 5, London, 1971, Heinemann Medical. Helpful and practical, the title of this book speaks for itself.

Morton, L.T.: Use of medical literature, ed. 2, Woburn, Mass., 1977, Butterworth
Publishers. This book's purpose is to provide a comprehensive guide to medical
literature, as well as sources of unpublished medical information. Seven chapters cover general aspects of information search and retrieval within specific
medical areas, including obstetrics and gynecology (Chapter 17).

National Library of Medicine audiovisuals catalog. An annotated list of 16 mm motion pictures and videotapes available from the National Medicine Audiovisuals
Center, Atlanta.

Psychological abstracts. Abstracts of books and articles in the social and behavioral
sciences arranged by subject matter.

Psychological Index. This is for the social and behavioral sciences what Index Medicus is for the medical sciences.

Sheehy, E.P., ed.: Guide to reference books, ed. 9, Chicago, 1976, American Library Association. The Reference Source of reference sources. Sometimes referred to as "Winchell," after the editor of the much-used 8th edition.

Sunners, W.: How and where to find the facts, New York, 1963, Arco Publishing, Inc. A helpful, general purpose book aptly described by its title. Chapter 3 focuses on how to use libraries.

Ubrich's international periodicals directory, ed. 20, New York, 1981, R.R. Bowker Co. Listing and brief description of periodicals within broad subject categories.

Union list of serials. Lists the periodical holdings of all libraries in the United States and Canada. Invaluable for interlibrary loan requests.

Wyner, B.S.: Reference books in paperback, ed. 2, Littleton, Colo., 1976, Libraries Unlimited, Inc. Lists the less expensive reference material sources. Indexing is by subject category as well as author and title.

Chapter 6

Alderson, G., and Sentman, E.: How you can influence congress: the complete handbook for the citizen lobbyist, New York, 1979, E.P. Dutton, Inc.

Annas, G.J.: Childbirth and the law: how to work within old laws, avoid malpractice, and influence new legislation in maternity care. In Stewart, D., and Stewart, L., eds.: 21st century obstetrics now! vol. 2, Marble Hill, Mo., 1977, NAPSAC Reproductions.

Annas, G.J.: Rights of hospital patients, New York, 1975, Avon Books.

Barasa, B.: Midwifery in court: attracting publicity. In Stewart, D., and Stewart, L., eds.: Compulsory hospitalization: freedom of choice in childbirth? vol. 2, Marble Hill, Mo., 1979, NAPSAC Reproductions.

Code of federal regulations. Codification of the general and permanent rules published in the Federal Register by the executive departments and agencies of the federal government. Each volume is revised at least once a year and issued quarterly.

Federal code of regulations, See Code of Federal Regulations.

Iffy, L., and Wecht, C.H.: Medical-legal aspects of perinatal and surgical infections. In Wecht, C.H., ed.: Legal medicine, Philadelphia, 1980, W.B. Saunders Co.

Katz, B.F.: Electronic fetal monitoring and the law, Birth Family J. 6(4):251, 1979.

Lander, L.: Defective medicine: risk, anger, and the malpractice crisis, New York, 1978, Farrar, Straus & Giroux, Inc.

The Law of Informed Consent. In President's Commission for the Study of Ethical Problems in Medicine and Biomedical and Behavioral Research, Making health care decisions: the ethical and legal implications of informed consent in the patient-practitioner relationship, vol. 3, Washington, D.C., October, 1982.

Law, S., and Polan, S.: Pain and profit: the politics of malpractice, New York, 1978, Harper & Row Publishers, Inc.

Midwifery and the law. This is an updated summary of each state's legislation regarding lay midwives. Issued by Mothering Publications, P.O. Box 2046, Albuquerque, N.M. 87103, as a separate or as part of Mothering Magazine's 1982 fall issue.

Pollack, R.S.: Clinical aspects of malpractice, Oradell, N.J., 1980, Medical Economics Books. This book was written for the physician. Available through Medical Economics Book Division, Box 157, Florence, Ky. 41042.

Stewart, D.: Informed consent. In Stewart, D., and Stewart, L., eds.: Compulsory hospitalization: freedom of choice in childbirth? vol. 3, Marble Hill, Mo., 1979, NAPSAC Reproductions.

Chapter 7

Childbirth choices: what to ask, where to go, who to see, Philadelphia, 1982, CHOICE. Write to CHOICE, 1501 Cherry St., Philadelphia, Pa. 19102.

Clavell, J., ed.: The art of war: Sun Tzu, New York, 1983, Delacorte Press.

Elkins, V.H.: The rights of the pregnant parent, rev. ed., New York, 1980, Schocken Books, Inc.

Fisher, R., and Ury, W.: Getting to yes, New York, 1983, Penguin Books.

Hornstein, F., and Waxman, J.G.: Birth rights: an advocate's guide to ending infant mortality, Los Angeles, 1983, National Health Law Program, Inc. (2639 South La Cienega Blvd., Los Angeles, Calif. 90034). Cost is $8.

McKay, S.: Assertive childbirth, Englewood Cliffs, N.J., 1983, Prentice-Hall, Inc.

Stewart, D., and Stewart, L., eds.: The childbirth activists' handbook, Marble Hill, Mo., 1983, NAPSAC Reproductions.

Young, D.: Changing childbirth: family birth in the hospital, Rochester, N.Y., 1982, Childbirth Graphics, Ltd.

Periodicals

Listed here are periodicals that frequently carry articles relating to health care and legal issues in pregnancy and childbirth.

American Journal of Law and Medicine. A quarterly publication that encompasses all aspects of medico-legal relations. It is published by the American Society of Law and Medicine and receives editorial support from Boston College of Law School and Boston University School of Law.

Birth. This is a quarterly publication sponsored by the International Childbirth Education Association and by the American Society for Psychoprophylaxis in Obstetrics. It is intended for the concerned provider and consumer of health care in childbearing. The journal's former name was *Birth and the Family Journal.*

ICEA News. Official quarterly publication of the International Childbirth Education Association. It provides information on family-centered birth alternatives, developments, meetings, and resources in the maternity and parenting fields. Available through ICEA, P.O. Box 20048, Minneapolis, Minn. 55420.

ICEA Review. Published three times a year, each issue examines a topic of current interest and/or controversy within the childbearing field, includes abstracts from literature as well as editorial and guest commentary. Available through ICEA, P.O. Box 20048, Minneapolis, Minn. 55420.

Law, Medicine and Health Care. A monthly publication that purports to consolidate medicolegal news with nursing law and ethics. It is published by the American Society of Law and Medicine.

Mothering. A quarterly magazine devoted to natural approaches to pregnancy, childbirth, midwifery, family health, and so forth. Available from Mothering Publications, Inc., P.O. Box 2046, Albuquerque, N.M. 87103.

NAPSAC News. Newsletter of InterNational Association of Parents and Professionals for Safe Alternatives in Childbirth. Available from NAPSAC Reproductions, P.O. Box 267, Marble Hill, Mo. 63764. NAPSAC is the largest and most active of the country's groups for parents.

Network News. The newsletter of the National Women's Health Network, published six times yearly. It provides members with legislative, political, and technological information on women's reproduction and general health. It is available for members of the NWHN, 224 7th St. S.E., Washington, D.C. 20003. Individual membership is $25.

Ob. Gyn. News. A semimonthly publication issued by International Medical News Group, 12230 Wilkins Ave., Rockville, Md. 20852. Billed as a "fast, accurate report" intended for obstetricians and gynecologists, it is nevertheless so clearly written and well edited that nonprofessionals can readily understand it.

The People's Doctor Newsletter. A bimonthly medical newsletter for consumers. Each issue highlights a specific medical area. Edited by Dr. Robert Mendelsohn. Available through The People's Doctor Newsletter, 664 N. Michigan Ave., Suite 720, Chicago, Il. 60611.

The Practicing Midwife. A quarterly newsletter published by The Farm, 156 Drakes Lane, Summertown, Tenn. 38483. It is for midwives and others interested in childbirth and health.

Women & Health. A quarterly journal directed toward health care professionals and health activists who are centrally concerned with women's issues in health care delivery. Available through Haworth Press, 28 East 22nd Street, New York, N.Y. 10010.

Films on Childbirth

Alternative Childbirth
This feature-length film depicts all the choices in childbirth available to couples today. Hospital, birth center, and home births (attended and unattended) are shown. Cinema Medica. 65 mins; color.

Anthony's Birth at Home
This film tells the story of a couple who, after being unable to find a medical attendant who would come to their home for her labor and delivery, decided to have the baby at home without medical supervision with the husband attending. Cinema Medica. 17 mins; color.

Birth
This film shows a natural childbirth using the Lamaze method. Filmakers Library. 40 mins; black and white.

Birth at Home
An Australian film that shows a home delivery assisted by a highly professional midwife who uses zonal massage and herbal medicine. Of special interest is the mother's unusual birthing position—on her hands and knees. This film does not advocate home over hospital birth, but shows a mother and her baby's needs being met in a relaxed and supportive environment. Filmakers Library. 14 mins; color.

Birth Centers
Parents and professionals give their views on birth centers, and couples are shown giving birth in them. Cinema Medica. 24 mins; color.

Birth in the Squatting Position
This is an incredible new film on an age-old method. Polymorph Films. 10 mins; color.

Birth Place
This film shows two families who share their birthing experiences with the viewer. Bureau of Audio Visual Instruction. 47 mins; color.

Cesarean Childbirth
This film shows that even in a surgical delivery many of the principles of family-centered maternity care can still be followed. Cinema Medica. 18 mins; color.

Childbirth
This is a documentary introduction to the birth of a baby. Polymorph Films. 17 mins; color.

Childbirth for the Joy of It, Part I
This film shows five couples giving birth with husbands in the delivery room and women delivering with minimum intervention. Cinema Medica. 23 mins; color.

Childbirth for the Joy of It, Part II
This film shows many of the advances made in family-centered maternity care. Cinema Medica. 24 mins; color.

Daughters of Time
This compelling film sensitively conveys the current trends in midwifery and the caring, competent women who are nurse-midwives. Durrin Films. 30 mins.

An Everyday Miracle—Birth
This is a documentary following the development of a baby from conception to birth. Microphotography provides pictures of a living human embryo within the womb. (From BBC) Films Incorporated.

Five Women Five Births
This film shows (1) alternative style birth in a hospital with an obstetrician; (2) natural birth in a home with family physician, Leboyer style; (3) unmedicated vaginal breech birth in a hospital with an obstetrician; (4) cesarean birth for breech in a hospital with an obstetrician; and (5) home birth with midwives, family, and friends. Suzanne Arms Productions. 29 mins; black and white.

Gentle Birth
This is a film of nonviolent childbirth with delivery and commentary by Dr. John Grover, who has adapted the pioneering work of Dr. Frederick Leboyer to American hospital practices. Polymorph Films. 15 mins; color.

Happy Birthday
The viewer experiences a delivery in a homelike hospital setting; the father's role is a major one. The woman delivers in a sitting position without stirrups. Cinema Medica. 17 mins; color.

Having a Section is Having a Baby
This film provides information about all aspects of cesarean delivery. Available as videocassette or as slide tray with audio cassette. Polymorph Films. 28 mins; color.

Midwife
This film is a documentary about two midwives showing their supportive involvement in two home births. Cinema Medica. 25 mins; color.

Midwife: With Woman
This is a straightforward, realistic, and inspiring account of nurse-midwives at work in a variety of down-to-earth situations. Fanlight Productions. 28 mins; color.

Not by Chance
This film depicts an attended home birth conducted according to the standards of the American College of Home Obstetrics. Cinema Medica. 22 mins; color.

Not me Alone
This film records one couple's labor and Lamaze type of delivery. Polymorph Films. 31 mins; color.

Obstetrical Intervention
This is a scientifically oriented film from a conference sponsored by the American Foundation for Maternal and Child Health; Dr. Roberto Caldeyro-Barcia, speaker. Cinema Medica. 43 mins; color.

Prenatal Diagnosis: to be or not to be
This film is about modern medicine's techniques that allow doctors to detect chemical abnormalities in utero. The presentation includes amniocentesis, fetoscopy, and ultrasound, as well as the birth defects that can be detected by these methods. Filmakers Library. 45 mins; color.

Primun non Nocere (Above All, Do No Harm)
This film shows a natural childbirth at home without anesthesia, analgesia, IV fluids, enema, shaving, stirrups, episiotomy, forceps, stitches, slapping of the baby, or separation of the baby from its parents. Cinema Medica. Color.

Saturday's Children
This film shows four prepared labors and births filmed during one remarkable Saturday. Featuring extraordinary birth sequences. Emphasizing labor-coaching techniques by partners and staff. Three primiparas, one multipara, one single mother. Parenting Pictures. 36 mins; color.

The Ties that Bind
A film portraying how relationships between parent and infant are experienced in pregnancy and during and immediately after birth. Polymorph Films. 27 mins; color.

When Life Begins
This film is a photographic depiction of prenatal development and an actual birth. Michigan State University Film Library. 14 mins; color.

Film Distributors

Bureau of Audio Visual Instruction, P.O. Box 2093, Madison, Wis. 53701, (608) 262-1644.

Cinema Medica (CMI), 2335 W. Foster Ave., Chicago, Ill. 60625, (312) 784-7686 (Illinois residents call collect). Out-of-state residents call (800) 621-5147.

Durrin Films, 1748 Kalorama Rd. N.W., Washington, D.C. 20009, (202) 966-2626.

Fanlight Productions, 47 Halifax St., Jamaica Plain, Mass. 02130, (617) 524-0980.

Filmakers Library, 290 West End Ave., New York, N.Y. 10023, (212) 355-6545.

Films Incorporated, 1144 Wilmette Ave., Wilmette, Ill. 60091, (800) 323-4222.

Michigan State University (MSU) Film Library, Instructional Media Center, East Lansing, Mich. 48824, (517) 353-3960.

Parenting Pictures, 121 NW Crystal St., Crystal River, Fla. 32629, (904) 795-2156.

Polymorph Films, 118 South St., Boston, Mass. 02111, (617) 542-2004.

Suzanne Arms Productions, 4370 Alpine, Portola Valley, Calif. 94301, (415) 851-8604.

C

Resource Organizations

Most of the following organizations were formed to help consumers and/or professionals by offering educational and informational services to childbearing families. Some do more than educate (see The Farm). For more detailed resource information, see NAPSAC's periodically updated Directory of Alternative Birth Services and Consumer Guide. The latest edition is available from NAPSAC Reproductions, P.O. Box 267, Marble Hill, Mo. 63764.

Alternative Birth Crisis Coalition, P.O. Box 48371, Chicago, IL 60648; (312) 625–4054. ABCC is a group of medical experts, with legal counsel, who specialize in defending physicians and midwives in legal difficulties regarding their licenses, hospital privileges, insurance, or criminal charges as a result of their involvement with home birth, birth centers, midwifery, or other alternatives to technological obstetrics.

American Academy of Husband-Coached Childbirth, P.O. Box 5224, Sherman Oaks, CA 91413; (213) 788–6662 or 788–6663. AAHCC trains and certifies childbirth educators in the Bradley method of natural childbirth.

American College of Home Obstetrics, P.O. Box 25, River Forest, IL 60305; (312) 383–1461. ACHO is a physician-sponsored organization whose purpose is to set standards for natural childbirth practice and for home obstetrics.

American College of Nurse-Midwives, 1522 K St. N.W., Suite 1120, Washington, DC 20005; (202) 347–5445. ACNM certifies nurse-midwives who practice in homes and hospitals and accredits education programs nationwide.

American Society for Psychoprophylaxis in Obstetrics, 1411 K Street N.W., Washington, DC 20005; (202) 783–7050. ASPO sponsors classes in the Lamaze method of prepared childbirth for expectant parents.

Association for Childbirth at Home, International, P.O. Box 39498, Los Angeles, CA 90039; (213) 667–0839. ACHI trains and certifies home birth teachers and midwives.

Cesarean Birth Alliance, 10 Summit Drive, Manhasset, NY 11030; (603) 435–6703, (617) 449–2490, or (617) 738–6750. CBA is a group of cesarean mothers who assist other mothers in avoiding unnecessary cesareans and who help mothers with previous cesareans to have vaginal births for subsequent births (vaginal birth after cesarean or VBAC). CBA also maintains a hotline for women who believe they are threatened by the prospect of a cesarean that may be unnecessary or who believe they have been subjected to an unnecessary cesarean.

Cesarean Prevention Movement, P.O. Box 152, Syracuse, NY 13210. Newly formed, CPM plans to function as a nationwide resource for information, education, and support for vaginal births after cesareans.

Cesareans/Support, Education, and Concern, 66 Christopher Road, Waltham, MA 02154; (617) 965–2781. C/SEC's purpose is to provide emotional and educational support for the cesarean parents by means of phone, correspondence, literature, audiovisual material, and hospital workshops.

Childbirth Without Pain Education Association, 20134 Snowden, Detroit, MI 48235; (313) 345–9850. CWPEA sponsors education and research in the psychoprophylactic method of painless childbirth.

The Farm, Summertown, TN 38483; (615) 964–3571. The Farm is a cooperative, village-style community of 1100. In 1971, it started developing a self-sufficient primary health care system, the most famous component of which is its midwife service. As of 1980, Farm midwives have delivered more than 1000 babies, at no charge to the parents. (Over half the women delivered at The Farm are not Farm members; mothers have come from as far away as Brazil to deliver there.) In the words of Ellen Brothers, Editor of *The Practicing Midwife*, a Farm periodical, "We feel that returning the major responsibility for normal childbirth to well-trained midwives rather than having it rest with profit-oriented, highly technological medical centers and hospitals is a major advance in self-determination for women."

Home Oriented Maternity Experience, Inc., 511 New York Avenue, Takoma Park, MD 20012; (301) 585–5832. HOME trains and certifies teachers for parents planning a home birth. HOME also organizes parent groups for mutual support and education in regard to home birth.

Informed Homebirth, Inc., P.O. Box 788, Boulder, CO 80306; (303) 444–0434. IH certifies home birth teachers and midwives. It offers a class series taught by its certified educators for couples planning a home birth. It also has a tape cassette course of self-instruction.

InterNational Association of Parents and Professionals for Safe Alternatives in Childbirth, P.O. Box 267, Marble Hill, MO 63764; (314) 238–2010. NAPSAC is dedicated to establishing family-centered childbirth programs for both in-hospital and out-of-hospital births, using both physicians and midwives. It sponsors major conferences and training workshops, publishes books, certifies maternity services, maintains a Directory of Alternative Birth Services, and produces a quarterly newsletter for its members. NAPSAC has access to attorneys and experts for defense of alternative birth parents and professionals.

International Childbirth Education Association, P.O. Box 20048, Minneapolis, MN 55420; (612) 854–8660. Family-centered care is ICEA's primary goal and the basis of ICEA philosophy. The concept of family-centered maternity care covers the entire childbearing period, from pregnancy to the adjustment of the new family unit. The concept is based on the needs of parents and families and on sound scientific evidence from medicine, sociology, psychology, nursing, midwifery, nutrition, and other fields. This integrated and individualized approach ensures total health care for the childbearing family—infant, parents, and siblings. ICEA endeavors to join together people interested in family-centered maternity and infant care to (1) promote education and preparation for childbearing, breastfeeding, and family-centered maternity care; (2) assist with the establishment of local groups with similar goals; and (3) further the understanding of ICEA's goals and philosophy by health providers and the general public. ICEA sponsors conferences and issues publications, including *ICEA Review, ICEA Forum,* and *ICEA Sharing.*

LaLeche League International, 9616 Minneapolis Ave., Franklin Park, IL 60131; (312) 455-7730. The LaLeche League is an organization of women devoted to better mothering through breastfeeding. It offers assistance to breastfeeding mothers and women considering breastfeeding through monthly meetings and telephone counseling services provided by local chapters of the International.

Midwives Alliance of North America, c/o Concord Midwifery Service, 30 S. Main St., Concord, NH 03301. MANA is an umbrella organization uniting midwives to build cooperation among them and to promote midwifery as a means of improving health care for women and their families.

NAPSAC: See "InterNational Association for Parents and Professionals for Safe Alternatives in Childbirth."

National Association for the Advancement of Leboyer's Birth Without Violence, NAALBWV National Headquarters, P.O. Box 248455, University of Miami Branch, Coral Gables, FL 33124; (305) 665-9506. NAALBWV sponsors education in the Leboyer approach to childbirth. The group informs the public and medical profession of this approach through films, discussions, and printed material. Articles are available free to members and for 40¢ per publication to nonmembers. Brochures and a description of available articles are free.

National Association of Childbearing Centers (formerly, Cooperative Birth Center Network), Box 1, Route 1, Perkiomenville, PA 18074; (215) 234-8068. The recently formed NACC assists and supports the development and accessibility of safe, cost-efficient birth alternatives, with particular attention to the out-of-hospital birth center.

National Association of Childbirth Education, 3940 11th Street, Riverside, CA 92501; (714) 686-0422. NACE sponsors education in the Pavlov-Lamaze method of childbirth.

National Center on Women and Family Law, 799 Broadway, Room 402, New York, NY 10003; (212) 674-8200. NCOWFL recently opened its family law library, one of the largest collections of material on family law in the country. The collection has material on women's health issues, child care, child abuse and neglect, statistics relating to women's issues, and other topics.

National Midwives Association, 1620 Howze Street, El Paso TX 79903; (915) 533-8142. NMA is an association of practicing midwives. Most members are lay midwives.

D

Midwives: How to Find One and What to Ask Her

Home birth becomes more popular every day. Between 1973 and 1980, home births increased 300%. Obstetricians and hospital administrators view this resurgence as a threat to their economic and power monopoly. In a desperate effort to turn the trend around, the medical community is trying to muscle midwives out of business (if not into jail). The net effect has been to drive midwives underground and make it more difficult for consumers to find them. The amount of detective work in "flushing out" a midwife depends on the state in which you live.

To locate a midwife, try one of the following links. Inquire at a woman's health center, at a childbirth group, at the local LaLeche League group, or at a freestanding birth center, if your community has one. Post notices on the bulletin boards of health food stores. Write ACHI, HOME, and NAP-SAC (see Appendix C) requesting names and phone numbers of midwives in your area. Sometimes, too, osteopaths and chiropractors know midwives and will refer you to them. Obtain a copy of the NAPSAC Directory of Alternative Birth Services, $5.95, from NAPSAC Reproductions, P.O. Box 267, Marble Hill, MO 63764. It lists over 2000 midwives with addresses and phone numbers.

Once you have found a midwife, here are some questions to ask her:

Are you a nurse-midwife or a lay (empirical) midwife?
Where and how were you trained?
How long have you been in practice?
How many out-of-hospital births have you attended? At home? At free-standing birth centers? For how many of these births have you been the *primary* attendant?

167

What is your philosophy about intervention in obstetrics?

What kind of childbirth instruction do you recommend or with what kind do you feel most comfortable? Are there any with which you feel uncomfortable?

Do you mind other people, including my other children, being present at the birth?

Do you provide prenatal care as well as delivery? Does delivery also include postnatal care?

What is your fee for prenatal care? For delivery and postnatal care?

Will my insurance pay for your services? (Some states, for example, Pennsylvania, have insurance laws permitting direct reimbursement of nurse-midwives.)

Do you bring an assistant to the birth? Who is your assistant and how skilled or experienced is he or she?

What equipment do you bring to the birth?

    1. Oxygen?

    2. Drugs or herbs? For what purpose?

    3. Pitocin or something to stop postpartum bleeding?

    4. Equipment for infant resuscitation?

Have you had experience in infant resuscitation?

Have you had experience in suturing?

Do you have a working relationship with a doctor in case I should need to see one during my pregnancy? In case of complications during delivery?

Is there a hospital that would take me in an emergency if I didn't have a private physician? Do you have a working relationship with that hospital so that you could come with me if complications developed and I had to deliver in-hospital?

What is your definition of an emergency requiring hospitalization?

Do you have a working relationship with paramedics?

Can you commit yourself to be free for my due date? What about early labor? What if you had an emergency of your own and couldn't make it? Who would deliver me then? Do you have a working relationship with other midwives in the community? How do I get in touch with you for something routine? For an emergency? How far away do you live?

E

Questions to Ask a Physician

Dr. Robert Mendelsohn advises that "The most important [thing] for your own protection is to ask the doctor questions. In some cases, he'll answer the questions. In most cases, the doctor will get upset. Ask the questions anyway."[1] Following each question are some points to consider in evaluating the physician's response. If the physician refuses to respond at all, run—don't walk—to the nearest exit!

How long have you been in practice?
Length of practice (and age) applies to your individual preferences. Some women prefer the older, more experienced physician to one who is still new to practice. Other women are looking for the younger physician who may be more willing to try new approaches.

How many babies have you delivered?
An older obstetrician may not be more experienced than a young one if he has recently switched to obstetrics from some other specialty area.

Will you deliver my baby at home?

At which hospital(s) do you practice?
Some physicians are affiliated with more than one hospital, but the bulk of a physician's practice will be at a single hospital. If, in your shopping around, you discover you do not like that hospital, you may want to change physicians. Choosing a physician and facility is not irreversible.

Are you board certified?
Board certified physicians are specialists in a particular area of medicine; they have successfully passed written and oral examinations that certify their expertise in this area. Board eligible means they have not yet taken written or oral exams but are eligible to do so. Being board certified or board eligible is reassuring but no guarantee of a physician's ability.

What is your fee for normal prenatal care and delivery?
Normal prenatal care (care during pregnancy) usually includes office visits and routine lab work (urinalysis, blood tests for protein and sugar levels, and antibody serum for the Rh factor). It will not cover the initial lab work-up (profile), which is a one-time fee, payable to the lab performing the tests. Usually included is a checkup 6 weeks after delivery.

What is your fee for a cesarean section?
This fee usually includes the prenatal visits, some lab work, the surgery itself, and postnatal visit(s). Often physicians order x-ray films or ultrasonography that are not included in their fees. The ultrasonography and x-ray films mean an additional professional fee, as well as a hospital fee for using the equipment.

Are payments required in advance of insurance reimbursement?
Re-read your insurance policy to determine what it will cover. Do not assume your insurance will cover everything! Your physician's office personnel will be able to tell you how to go about filing your claim. Many physicians require payment in full by the seventh month although insurance companies will not reimburse until the baby is born. (Remember, the physician's fee is separate from the hospital's fee, which will also be due at the same time.) Physicians' financial practices vary. Their receptionists will usually be willing to give you specific information over the telephone.

Do you and your hospital encourage prepared childbirth? Family-centered childbirth? Neither?
Almost all hospitals now offer some variety of support for prepared childbirth, but not all physicians support it. "Prepared childbirth" generally means the mother and father have participated in a course in childbirth. "Family-centered care" is a relatively new concept that incorporates all the aspects of prepared childbirth but goes a step further by trying to provide a homelike environment within the hospital, for example, regular beds, lamps, windows, chairs, and curtains, rather than hospital beds, tiled walls, and stainless steel. The hospital may call this their "birthing room." The goal of family-centered care is to make the birthing a family event to be celebrated with as little medical intervention as possible. The baby is allowed to stay with the mother during her entire stay, which is usually brief (6 to 12 hours).

Do you encourage breastfeeding?
Breastfeeding is now recognized as the feeding method of choice for both physiological and psychological reasons. If you choose to breastfeed, it is best to know as much as possible before you put your baby to the breast. It is a learned art and, until recently, an almost lost art. It will require determination on your part and support from those around you. Most physicians seem to have a very limited understanding of the process and can be

of little help in the how-to department. However, if you know your physician will be supportive, it could make a difference should you get sick or develop a breast infection. LaLeche League International is an organization of women devoted to better mothering through breastfeeding. Local groups hold monthly meetings and offer telephone counseling. They are experts in this area and will be happy to give you information on the subject.

Which of the following do you routinely incorporate into your practice?
During pregnancy

Amniocentesis is a procedure for removing a sample of amniotic fluid to test for fetal abnormalities, fetal maturity, and fetal sex. A long needle is inserted through the abdomen, into the uterus, and into the amniotic sac, where the fetus is floating in amniotic fluid. A portion of the fluid is withdrawn. Laboratory tests of the fluid can determine such things as Down's syndrome and the sex of the child. As with all medical procedures, there is a certain risk involved. In this case, a chief risk is hitting the fetus or placenta with the needle. In addition to the risk of death, a British study found amniocentesis to be associated with increased rates of maternal antepartum hemorrhage, neonatal respiratory distress, and major orthopedic deformities.[2] Finally, amniocentesis is painful.

Despite the risks and despite the lack of compelling reasons for making amniocentesis a routine procedure, some obstetricians perform an amniocentesis on most of their patients. As one mother reported,

> Amniocentesis is done routinely by all OB's in this area to determine if a baby is ready to be born C-Section. My friend was expecting her fourth child [and] her OB did an amniocentesis on her to find out if her baby was "ready" to be taken C-section.

> The reason her OB did the amniocentesis was because he was leaving on vacation and wanted to do her C-section himself. In the process of doing the amniocentesis, he did much damage to her baby. The child weighed 7 pounds 1 ounce at birth but died at 6 days. The autopsy report (which they tried to keep from the parents) stated that the baby died from stress. It was their only girl.

> It seems the doctor had told them that the amniocentesis was a perfectly harmless procedure.

> The doctor attempted four times to obtain adequate fluid while his nurse pushed up on the baby's head from her vagina and the doctor pushed on the baby externally. The fourth time he broke her water while extracting fluid.[3]

Diuretics, also known as water pills, used to be widely prescribed to relieve swelling. Swelling is normal in all pregnant mammals. The FDA now frowns on the use of diuretics as both useless and unsafe in reducing the normal swelling of pregnancy (except for women with high blood pressure and certain forms of heart disease). The FDA also frowns on the practice of urging women to be extremely careful about their weight gain. Using diuretics and restricting weight gain can set the stage for a condition called toxemia, an indication for a surgical delivery.[4]

Dieting to control weight.
Vitamin supplements.

Ultrasonography is a relatively new diagnostic technique that is replacing x-ray films. It uses sound waves to create a picture of the abdominal area. It is used as an aid in amniocentesis and can spot placenta previa. It can also help determine the age of the fetus. Many physicians have their patients undergo this procedure to determine expected due date. We remind you that this is a new technique whose possible side effects and risks have not been fully assessed.

During labor and delivery (See Chapter 1 for a discussion of these points.)
Shaving.
Enemas.
Fasting.
Intravenous "feeding."
Induction.
Electronic fetal monitoring.
Horizontal position.
Frequent vaginal exams.
Episiotomy.
Analgesic painkillers or other preanesthetic medication.
Local anesthetic.
General anesthetic.
Forceps or other mechanical means of extracting the baby.

Nursing on the delivery table is something you may not care about if you do not intend to continue to breastfeed. However, many regard it as very important. Early nursing enhances the development of the bonding process between mother and child and stimulates the letdown reflex for the production of milk. Milk does not come in right away, but colostrum does. It is a yellowish fluid that contains many immunities that are passed from mother to baby. Your baby will not get these immunities any other way. Immediate sucking at the breast also stimulates hormone production in the mother, which speeds placental expulsion and uterine shrinkage.

Sibling visitation after the baby is born.

Early release from the hospital (12 to 24 hours) is a growing trend among couples who want to lessen the psychological, physiological, and financial stress of hospitalization. Talk this over with your pediatrician as well.

Under what circumstances would you elect to perform a cesarean section? (See Chapter 1.)

What is your cesarean section rate? (See Chapter 1.)

Do residents or interns assist in your practice?
Very often residents or interns will assist physicians in their practices. You have a right to know if your physician supervises a resident or intern. You may refuse treatment from anyone you do not know (or, for that matter, anyone you know). Residents and interns are not as experienced as your own physician. In reality, they are apprentices.

Who are your partners? Do they share your philosophies? If no partners, who covers for you?
Make a point of meeting your physician's partners or those who cover for your physician. Your own physician will not be able to attend the delivery of every patient seen during her pregnancy. Make sure the partners and covering physicians share the same philosophies as your own physician. If not, when you check into the hospital and find the partner on duty, you will either face a big disappointment or an unpleasant clash of wills. In neither case will you have a joyful experience.

Do you have a midwife on your staff?
An increasing number of obstetricians are adding midwives to their staffs. They typically deal with women whose pregnancies are progressing normally. Many patients find that midwives are superior to their obstetrician employers in providing warmth, understanding, attentiveness, information, and flexibility in matters to be negotiated.

Do you and the hospital allow fathers in the labor room? in the delivery room? to be present during cesarean sections?
Mothers need a support person and fathers need to bond.

Do you and the hospital allow siblings to visit the baby?

What is your view on circumcision? Do you do it yourself or allow students to do it? What is your fee?
Circumcision removes the foreskin from the end of the penis by surgical or other means. The boy's health does not require circumcision. Rather, it is a custom in the United States, where most males are circumcised. (In England, on the other hand, less than 1% of male babies are circumcised.) Circumcision is usually done by the physician, though sometimes by students, shortly after birth. The fee is in addition to the physician's delivery

charge. You should decide whether you want your boy circumcised before you go into the hospital.

What methods of contraception do you recommend?
Most physicians will bring up the subject if you don't. Pregnancy puts a great deal of stress on even the healthiest of bodies, so it is a good idea to space your children. None of the methods is 100% effective, and all have some side effects or drawbacks. The pill is out if you are breastfeeding.

Do you do tubal ligation? What is your fee?
The charges for tubal ligation (sterilization) are highest when it is done as an independent procedure, intermediate when it is done at time of vaginal delivery, and lowest when it is done during cesarean section.

This is a permanent sterilization procedure that can sometimes be reversed by surgery. Since it is a surgical procedure, it will be necessary for you to sign a consent form. Don't wait to sign such an agreement until you are under the stress of labor and influence of drugs. Discuss sterilization with your physician before you deliver. If you decide to have it done at the time of your delivery, discuss with your physician the possibility that you may want a release from your agreement if something is wrong with your baby. You can always have it done later.

More step-by-step advice on how to interview an obstetrician can be found in Sheila Kitzinger's *The Complete Book of Pregnancy and Childbirth* (New York, 1980, Alfred A. Knopf, Inc.)

Notes
1. Mendelsohn, R.: Confessions of a medical heretic, Chicago, 1979, Contemporary Books, Inc., p. 44.
2. Medical Research Council Report in a Special Supplement to the Br. J. Obstet. Gynaecol., **86**:1–3, February 1979.
3. Letter to NAPSAC from Donna Schumacher, Kimberly, Wisconsin, Reprinted by permission from NAPSAC News, **6**(4):15, 1981.
4. Randall, J.: Too many cesareans? Parents Mag., p. 72, November 1978.

F

Sample Patient-Doctor Contract

All of the preferences listed below presume normal birth conditions. In the event of medical emergency or need, we agree to accept medical judgments with informed consent. The items checked below indicate our preferences.

Generally

____ Clear and adequate explanations of procedures, progress, and complications

____ Baby's father present

____ Photographs

____ All personnel introduced to us by name and position

____ Respect for our privacy

Labor

____ Mini or no prep (shave)

____ To walk around freely during labor (before water breaks)

____ Vaginal exams only with explanation, permission, and after appropriate introduction by examiner

____ Companion present during all examinations and procedures

____ IV only if necessary

____ Fetal heart monitor only if necessary, for specific reasons explained thoroughly

____ A monitrice (labor coach) in addition to father or companion

____ More than one companion, for example, father and friend

____ Beverages during labor

____ No artificial rupture of membranes (unless medically indicated)

Drugs

____ No analgesia (Demerol, Nisentil, and the like) unless we request it

____ No anesthesia (peridural, caudal, spinal, general, and the like) unless we request it

____ No stimulation or induction of labor (unless medically indicated)

Delivery

____ Freedom to choose position for birth

____ Backrest on delivery table

____ No wrist or leg restraints

____ No stirrups/low stirrups

____ No sterile drapes

____ Mirror (positioned for mother to watch baby's birth)

____ No routine episiotomy

____ Quiet at birth

____ Immediate skin-to-skin contact with baby

____ Delayed clamping of umbilical cord, until pulsation ceases

____ Hold baby immediately

____ Warm bath for baby

Adapted from the Childbirth Preferences List, Consumers for Choices in Childbirth, P.O. Box 24, Guilford, CT 06437. With permission.

G

Patient's Bill of Rights

The American Hospital Association presents a Patient's Bill of Rights with the expectation that observance of these rights will contribute to more effective patient care and greater satisfaction for the patient, his physician, and the hospital organization. Further, the Association presents these rights in the expectation that they will be supported by the hospital on behalf of its patients, as an integral part of the healing process. It is recognized that a personal relationship between the physician and the patient is essential for the provision of proper medical care. The traditional physician-patient relationship takes on a new dimension when care is rendered within an organizational structure. Legal precedent has established that the institution itself also has a responsibility to the patient. It is in recognition of these factors that these rights are affirmed.

1. The patient has the right to considerate and respectful care.
2. The patient has the right to obtain from his physician complete current information concerning his diagnosis, treatment, and prognosis in terms the patient can be reasonably expected to understand. When it is not medically advisable to give such information to the patient, the information should be made available to an appropriate person in his behalf. He has the right to know, by name, the physician responsible for coordinating his care.
3. The patient has the right to receive from his physician information necessary to give informed consent prior to the start of any procedure and/or treatment. Except in emergencies, such information for informed consent should include but not necessarily be limited to the specific procedure and/or treatment, the medically significant risks involved, and the probable duration of incapacitation. Where

From *A Patient's Bill of Rights*, published by the American Hospital Association, copyright 1975.

medically significant alternatives for care or treatment exist, or when the patient requests information concerning medical alternatives, the patient has the right to such information. The patient also has the right to know the name of the person responsible for the procedures and/or treatment.

4. The patient has the right to refuse treatment to the extent permitted by law and to be informed of the medical consequences of his action.

5. The patient has the right to every consideration of his privacy concerning his own medical care program. Case discussion, consultation, examination, and treatment are confidential and should be conducted discreetly. Those not directly involved in his care must have the permission of the patient to be present.

6. The patient has the right to expect that all communications and records pertaining to his care should be treated as confidential.

7. The patient has the right to expect that within its capacity a hospital must make reasonable response to the request of a patient for services. The hospital must provide evaluation, service, and/or referral as indicated by the urgency of the case. When medically permissible, a patient may be transferred to another facility only after he has received complete information and explanation concerning the needs for and alternatives to such a transfer. The institution to which the patient is to be transferred must first have accepted the patient for transfer.

8. The patient has the right to obtain information as to any relationship of his hospital to other health care and educational institutions insofar as his care is concerned. The patient has the right to obtain information as to the existence of any professional relationships among individuals, by name, who are treating him.

9. The patient has the right to be advised if the hospital proposes to engage in or perform human experimentation affecting his care or treatment. The patient has the right to refuse to participate in such research projects.

10. The patient has the right to expect reasonable continuity of care. He has the right to know in advance what appointment times and physicians are available and where. The patient has the right to expect that the hospital will provide a mechanism whereby he is informed by his physician or a delegate of the physician of the patient's continuing health care requirements following discharge.

11. The patient has the right to examine and receive an explanation of his bill regardless of source of payment.

12. The patient has the right to know what hospital rules and regulations apply to his conduct as a patient.

No catalog of rights can guarantee for the patient the kind of treatment he has a right to expect. A hospital has many functions to perform, including the prevention and treatment of disease, the education of both health professionals and patients, and the conduct of clinical research. All these activities must be conducted with an overriding concern for the patient and, above all, the recognition of his dignity as a human being. Success in achieving this recognition assures success in the defense of the rights of the patient.

H

The Pregnant Patient's Bill of Rights
The Pregnant Patient's Responsibilities

American parents are becoming increasingly aware that well-intentioned health professionals do not always have scientific data to support common American obstetrical practices and that many of these practices are carried out primarily because they are part of medical and hospital tradition. In the last forty years many artificial practices have been introduced which have changed childbirth from a physiological event to a very complicated medical procedure in which all kinds of drugs are used and procedures carried out, sometimes unnecessarily, and many of them potentially damaging for the baby and even for the mother. A growing body of research makes it alarmingly clear that every aspect of traditional American hospital care during labor and delivery must now be questioned as to its possible effect on the future well-being of both the obstetric patient and her unborn child.

One in every 35 children born in the United States today will eventually be diagnosed as retarded; in 75% of these cases there is no familial or genetic predisposing factor. One in every 10 to 17 children has been found to have some form of brain dysfunction or learning disability requiring special treatment. Such statistics are not confined to the lower socioeconomic group but cut across all segments of American society.

Reprinted with permission of Doris Haire, American Foundation for Maternal and Child Health; consultant, International Childbirth Education Association.

New concerns are being raised by childbearing women because no one knows what degree of oxygen depletion, head compression, or traction by forceps the unborn or newborn infant can tolerate before that child sustains permanent brain damage or dysfunction. The recent findings regarding the cancer-related drug diethylstilbestrol have alerted the public to the fact that neither the approval of a drug by the U.S. Food and Drug Administration nor the fact that a drug is prescribed by a physician serves as a guarantee that a drug or medication is safe for the mother or her unborn child. In fact, the American Academy of Pediatrics' Committee on Drugs has recently stated that there is no drug, whether prescription or over-the-counter remedy, which has been proven safe for the unborn child.

The Pregnant Patient has the right to participate in decisions involving her well-being and that of her unborn child, unless there is a clearcut medical emergency that prevents her participation. In addition to the rights set forth in the American Hospital Association's "Patient's Bill of Rights" (which has also been adopted by the New York City Department of Health), the Pregnant Patient, because she represents TWO patients rather than one, should be recognized as having the additional rights listed below.

1. *The Pregnant Patient has the right*, prior to the administration of any drug or procedure, to be informed by the health professional caring for her of any potential direct or indirect effects, risks or hazards to herself or her unborn or newborn infant which may result from the use of a drug or procedure prescribed for or administered to her during pregnancy, labor, birth or lactation.

2. *The Pregnant Patient has the right*, prior to the proposed therapy, to be informed, not only of the benefits, risks and hazards of the proposed therapy but also of known alternative therapy, such as available childbirth education classes which could help to prepare the Pregnant Patient physically and mentally to cope with the discomfort or stress of pregnancy and the experience of childbirth, thereby reducing or eliminating her need for drugs and obstetric intervention. She should be offered such information early in her pregnancy in order that she may make a reasoned decision.

3. *The Pregnant Patient has the right*, prior to the administration of any drug, to be informed by the health professional who is prescribing or administering the drug to her that any drug which she receives during pregnancy, labor and birth, no matter how or when the drug is taken or administered, may adversely affect her unborn baby, directly or indirectly, and that there is no drug or chemical which has been proven safe for the unborn child.

4. *The Pregnant Patient has the right*, if Cesarean section is anticipated, to be informed prior to the administration of any drug, and preferably prior to her hospitalization, that minimizing her

and, in turn, her baby's intake of nonessential preoperative medicine will benefit her baby.

5. *The Pregnant Patient has the right*, prior to the administration of a drug or procedure, to be informed of the areas of uncertainty if there is NO properly controlled follow up research which has established the safety of the drug or procedure with regard to its direct and/or indirect effects on the physiological, mental and neurological development of the child exposed, via the mother, to the drug or procedure during pregnancy, labor, birth or lactation (this would apply to virtually all drugs and the vast majority of obstetric procedures).

6 . *The Pregnant Patient has the right*, prior to the administration of any drug, to be informed of the brand name and generic name of the drug in order that she may advise the health professional of any past adverse reaction to the drug.

7 . *The Pregnant Patient has the right* to determine for herself, without pressure from her attendant, whether she will accept the risks inherent in the proposed therapy or refuse a drug or procedure.

8. *The Pregnant Patient has the right* to know the name and qualifications of the individual administering a medication or procedure to her during labor or birth.

9. *The Pregnant Patient has the right* to be informed, prior to the administration of any procedure, whether that procedure is being administered to her for her or her baby's benefit (medically indicated) or as an elective procedure (for convenience, teaching purposes or research).

10. *The Pregnant Patient has the right* to be accompanied during the stress of labor and birth by someone she cares for, and to whom she looks for emotional comfort and encouragement.

11. *The Pregnant Patient has the right* after appropriate medical consultation to choose a position for labor and for birth which is least stressful to her baby and to herself.

12. *The Obstetric Patient has the right* to have her baby cared for at her bedside if the baby is normal, and to feed her baby according to her baby's needs rather than according to the hospital regimen.

13. *The Obstetric Patient has the right* to be informed in writing of the name of the person who actually delivered her baby and the professional qualifications of that person. This information should also be on the birth certificate.

14. *The Obstetric Patient has the right* to be informed if there is any known or indicated aspect of her baby's care or condition which may cause her or her baby later difficulty or problems.

15. *The Obstetric Patient has the right* to have her and her baby's hospital medical records complete, accurate and legible and to have their records, including nursing notes, and to receive a

copy upon payment of a reasonable fee and without incurring the expense of retaining an attorney.

16. *The Obstetric Patient*, both during and after her hospital stay, has the right to have access to her complete hospital medical records, including nursing notes, and to receive a copy upon payment of a reasonable fee and without incurring the expense of retaining an attorney.

It is the obstetric patient and her baby, not the health professional, who must sustain any trauma or injury resulting from the use of a drug or obstetric procedure. The observation of the rights listed will not only permit the obstetric patient to participate in the decisions involving her and her baby's health care, but will help to protect the health professional and the hospital against litigation arising from resentment or misunderstanding on the part of the mother.

In addition to understanding her rights, the Pregnant Patient should also understand that she too has certain responsibilities. The Pregnant Patient's responsibilities include the following:

1. The Pregnant Patient is responsible for learning about the physical and psychological process of labor, birth and postpartum recovery. The better informed expectant parents are, the better they will be able to participate in decisions concerning the planning of their care.

2. The Pregnant Patient is responsible for learning what comprises good prenatal and intranatal care and for making an effort to obtain the best care possible.

3. Expectant parents are responsible for knowing about those hospital policies and regulations which will affect their birth and postpartum experience.

4. The Pregnant Patient is responsible for arranging for a companion or support person (husband, mother, sister, friend, etc.) who will share in her plans for birth and who will accompany her during her labor and birth experience.

5. The Pregnant Patient is responsible for making her preferences known clearly to the health professionals involved in her case in a courteous and cooperative manner and for making mutually agreed upon arrangements regarding maternity care alternatives with her physician or hospital in advance of labor.

6. Expectant parents are responsible for listening to their chosen physician or midwife with an open mind, just as they expect him or her to listen openly to them.

7. Once they have agreed to a course of health care, expectant parents are responsible, to the best of their ability, for seeing that the program is carried out in consultation with others with whom they have made the agreement.

8. The Pregnant Patient is responsible for obtaining information

in advance regarding the approximate cost of her obstetric and
hospital care.

9. The Pregnant Patient who intends to change her physician or
hospital is responsible for notifying all concerned, well in advance of the birth if possible, and for informing both of her
reasons for changing.

10. In all their interactions with medical and nursing personnel,
the expectant parents should behave toward those caring for
them with the same respect and consideration they themselves
would like.

11. During the mother's hospital stay, the mother is responsible for
learning about her and her baby's continuing care after discharge from the hospital.

12. After birth, the parents should put into writing constructive
comments and feelings of satisfaction and/or dissatisfaction
with the care (nursing, medical, and personal) they received.
Good service to families in the future will be facilitated by those
parents who take the time and responsibility to write letters expressing their feelings about the maternity care they received.

All the previous statements assume a normal birth and postpartum experience. Expectant parents should realize that, if complications develop in
their cases, there will be an increased need to trust the expertise of the
physician and hospital staff they have chosen. However, if problems occur, the childbearing woman still retains her responsibility for making informed decisions about her care or treatment and that of her baby. If she
is incapable of assuming that responsibility because of her physical condition, her previously authorized companion or support person should
assume responsibility for making informed decisions on her behalf.

I

Questions to Ask a Hospital

The cost of having a baby is expensive. Unlike the physician's fee, which is usually fixed for normal delivery, fees for hospital care are subject to many variables. Some hospitals charge for even a few minutes' use of the labor room, whereas others charge only after extended use. Delivery room fees may be a flat rate or broken down to half-hour intervals. These fees will also depend on the type of delivery, including equipment and supplies. Since it is major surgery, a cesarean section will greatly increase your hospital costs.

Ask the hospital administrator (or your physician) what the cesarean-section rate is for that hospital. Rates vary among hospitals, just as they vary among physicians. For example, among upstate New York hospitals in 1977, surgical delivery rates ranged from 1% to 23%.[1] For the country as a whole, cesarean-section rates have generally been lowest for small hospitals, that is, hospitals with fewer than 300 beds or 5000 annual discharges.

Generally, hospital room rates include three meals a day, nursing care, and a supply of personal care items, such as sanitary napkins. As a rule, if you request something that is not in your room, it will be charged to your bill.

Additional questions to ask about costs include the hospital's daily or one-time charges for the following: labor room, delivery room, operating room, recovery room, bed on ward, semiprivate room, private room, and electronic fetal monitor. (You may even be charged by the roll for the print-out paper the monitor uses.)

You may not realize that there is also a charge for the nursery, usually a flat daily rate. Should the baby require intensive care, the cost increases considerably. Baby supplies, diapers, soap, and formula are generally part of the standard nursery fee.

185

Early discharge can greatly decrease your bill. If you and your baby are doing well and you would like to go home, discuss it with your physician. You can, of course, leave at any time. However, if you leave against medical advice, your insurance company may balk at paying your charges.

If you have health insurance, find your policy and determine exactly what it covers. For example, if an anesthetic is administered to you by your physician rather than by an anesthesiologist, your insurance may not cover the physician's fee for that service. Also, some insurance companies will not cover a newborn until it is a specified age. If the baby dies before it reaches that age, the insurance will not pay the nursery fees.

If you have no insurance or only limited coverage, the hospital will probably want a large down payment by your seventh month of pregnancy. Contact the hospital's financial advisor to work out a payment arrangement. However, do not wait until your seventh month to do this or you may find that the hospital will not admit you.

When you get your bill, remember that anything the physician has ordered specifically for you or your baby will be an extra charge. These items will generally appear on your computerized bill under the heading of "drugs" with a code number, followed by the unit price. If you have a question about your bill, call the billing office and ask for a breakdown of the codes. Usually the bill you receive upon leaving the hospital is only an estimate. The final bill will be mailed to you within a few weeks.

Note

1. Fleck, A.: Personal communication.

Appendix

J

Consent Form and Medical Records

Consent Form

Request a copy of the consent form required to be signed by obstetrical patients before they are admitted to the hospital. After reviewing the consent form with a sympathetic physician and attorney, the attorney could then ask to meet with the hospital administrator, the hospital attorney, and the chief of obstetrics, to develop a consent form that will not only protect the patient but also protect the hospital and doctor. (A consent form that deals honestly with the risks, hazards, and pertinent areas of uncertainty, as well as the benefits of a treatment or procedure, can help to protect everyone.)

Patient Acquisition of Hospital Medical Records

Some hospitals destroy the medical records shortly after the patient leaves. Others keep them for a limited time and then dispose of them.

If you would like to obtain a copy of your hospital medical records, it is more effective if the letter shown here is sent to the chief administrator of the hospital. To get the name, call the hospital and ask for the "Administrator's Office." Tell the secretary that you would like to address a letter to the chief administrative officer and would like that person's name and official title. Such information is usually readily given.

Make several copies of the letter you send. Send a follow-up copy of your letter in 2 weeks if you have not received a reply. If you have not re-

Reprinted with permission from Stewart, D., and Stewart, L., eds.: 21st century obstetrics now! vol. 2, Marble Hill, Mo., 1977, NAPSAC Reproductions, and the American Foundation for Maternal and Child Health.

ceived your medical records or a satisfactory reply within 1 month of sending the first letter, you may choose to send the second, less friendly letter. The word "authorize" in the letter is essential.

Address
Date

Chief Administrative Officer
_____ Hospital
Our Town, U.S.A. 00000

Dear Sir:

I hereby authorize the administration of (*name of hospital*) to release directly to me a copy of my and my baby's complete hospital medical records, including nursing notes, pertaining to our stay in _____ Hospital from <u>date</u> to <u>date</u>. I will pay an appropriate fee for the reproduction of our records and for first-class postage.

I realize that the physical records belong to the hospital; however, I am aware that the information contained in our records belongs to me. I therefore authorize the administration of _____ Hospital to send a complete copy of my and my baby's complete records, including nursing notes, directly to me, not to my doctor. I wish to maintain a copy of my and my baby's complete hospital medical records in my own files and would appreciate a friendly compliance with my request.

Sincerely,

Ms. Jane Smith

Address
Date

Chief Administrative Officer
_____ Hospital
Our Town, U.S.A. 00000

Dear Sir:

In my letter of <u>date</u> (see enclosed copy) I requested that you release directly to me a copy of my and my baby's complete hospital medical records, including nursing notes, pertaining to our stay in ____ _____ Hospital from <u>date</u> to <u>date</u>. I have authorized the release of our records directly to me (not to my doctor) and have offered to pay an appropriate fee for their reproduction and mailing by first-class mail. Your refusal to comply with my request indicates either that you and your hospital have something to hide or that I have not stated my authorization properly. If the latter is the cause for the delay, I would appreciate your advising me as to the proper procedure for securing the records I have requested.

If I do not receive a complete copy of our hospital medical records (I do not wish a summary or extract) within 2 weeks, you will force me to bring legal action against the hospital to obtain our records.

It would be foolish indeed if the hospital forces me to take legal action when mere compliance with my request would solve the problem in an amicable way.

Sincerely,

Ms. Jane Smith

In the event that the hospital proposes to charge you more than 15¢ or 25¢ a page, ask the hospital's Medical Record Administrator what the copying charge is per page when hospital records are requested by a physician. There is no justification for the charges to be different—a patient's retention of a copy of his or her hospital records ensures continuity of care. If the hospital persists in charging you a higher rate, contact your local newspaper's health editor and suggest that the newspaper publicize this obvious effort to place obstacles in the way of patients' access to their own medical records.

Index